Fat removal

Fat removal

Invasive and non-invasive body contouring

Mathew M. Avram MD, JD

Dermatology Laser & Cosmetic Center
Massachusetts General Hospital
Boston, MA, USA

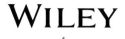

This edition first published 2015; © 2015 by John Wiley & Sons Ltd

Registered office: John Wiley & Sons, Ltd, The Atrium, Southern Gate, Chichester, West Sussex, PO19 8SQ, UK

Editorial offices: 9600 Garsington Road, Oxford, OX4 2DQ, UK
111 River Street, Hoboken, NJ 07030-5774, USA

For details of our global editorial offices, for customer services and for information about how to apply for permission to reuse the copyright material in this book please see our website at www.wiley.com/wiley-blackwell

Library of Congress Cataloging-in-Publication Data

Fat removal : invasive and non-invasive body contouring / [edited by] Mathew M. Avram.
    p. ; cm.
  Includes bibliographical references and index.
    ISBN 978-1-4443-3428-9 (cloth)
  I. Avram, Mathew M., editor.
  [DNLM: 1. Lipectomy–methods. 2. Adipose Tissue–surgery. WO 600]
  RD119.5.L55
  617.9′52–dc23

                                  2014035664

A catalogue record for this book is available from the British Library.

Wiley also publishes its books in a variety of electronic formats. Some content that appears in print may not be available in electronic books.

Typeset in 9.5/13pt MeridienLTStd by Laserwords Private Limited, Chennai, India

1 2015

Contents

List of contributors

Kenneth Arndt MD
President, SkinCare Physicians, Chestnut
Hill, MA, USA
Clinical Professor of Dermatology Emeritus,
Harvard Medical School, Boston, MA, USA
Adjunct Professor of Dermatology, Brown
University, Providence, RI, USA
Adjunct Professor, Department of Surgery,
The Geisel School of Medicine at Dartmouth,
Hanover, NH, USA

Alison Avram MD
Dermatology Laser & Cosmetic Center,
Massachusetts General Hospital, Boston, MA,
USA

Mathew M. Avram, MD
Dermatology Laser & Cosmetic Center,
Massachusetts General Hospital, MA,
USA

Suveena Bhutani MD
Sadick Dermatology and Research, NY, USA

Rebecca Fitzgerald MD
Division of Dermatology, David Geffen
School of Medicine, University of California,
Los Angeles (UCLA), Los Angeles, CA,
USA
Private Practice, Los Angeles, CA, USA

Selim M. Nasser MD
Department of Pathology, Clemenceau
Medical Center, Beirut, Lebanon

Andrew A. Nelson MD
Nelson Dermatology, Saint Petersburg, FL,
USA
Assistant Clinical Professor, Department of
Dermatology, Tufts University School of
Medicine, Boston, MA, USA

Arisa E. Ortiz MD
Director, Laser and Cosmetic Surgery,
Assistant Clinical Professor, Division of
Dermatology, University of California, San
Diego, USA

H. H. Ray Jalian MD
Division of Dermatology, David Geffen
School of Medicine, University of California,
Los Angeles (UCLA), Los Angeles, CA, USA

Adam M. Rotunda MD, FAAD, FACMS
Assistant Clinical Professor, Division of
Dermatology, David Geffen School of
Medicine, University of California Los
Angeles (UCLA), Los Angeles, CA, USA

**Neil S. Sadick MD, FAAD, FAACS,
FACP, FACPh**
Clinical Professor, Weill Cornell Medical
College, Cornell University, New York, NY,
USA

Nazanin Saedi MD
Assistant Professor, Director, Laser Surgery
and Cosmetic Dermatology, Department of
Dermatology and Cutaneous Biology,
Thomas Jefferson University, Philadelphia,
PA, USA

Zeina S. Tannous MD
Department of Dermatology, Massachusetts
General Hospital, Harvard Medical School,
Boston, MA, USA

Robert A. Weiss MD
Clinical Associate Professor, Department of
Dermatology, University of Maryland School
of Medicine, Baltimore, MD, USA
Director, MD Laser Skin Vein Institute,
Baltimore, MD, USA

Abbreviations

ACE	Angiotensin I converting enzyme
AGT	Angiotensinogen
AMP	Adenosine monophosphate
AR	Andrenergic receptor
ASAL	American Society for Aesthetic Lipodissolve
ATP	Adenosine triphosphate
β-AR	Beta-adrenergic receptors
BAT	Brown adipocyte tissue
BMI	Body mass index
BSA	Bovine serum albumin
CaHA	Calcium hydroxylapatite
CF	Central forehead
cGMP	Current Good Manufacturing Practice
CIF	Cooling intensity factor
CW	Continuous wave
DMCF	Deep medial cheek fat
EBP	Enhanced-binding protein
ELOS	Electro-Optical Synergy
EN	Erythema nodosum
EPAT	Extracorporeal Pulse Activation Technology
FDA	U.S. Food and Drug Administration
FFA	Free fatty acids
GAG	Glycosaminoglycan
GAIS	Global Aesthetic Improvement Score
HA	Hyaluronic acid
HAART	Highly active antiretroviral therapy
HDL	High-density lipoprotein
HIF1A	Hypoxia-inducible factor-1 alpha
HSL	Hormone sensitive lipase
IL-6	Interleukin-6
IO	Infraorbital
IR	Infrared
IRB	
LAL	Laser-assisted liposuction
LO	Lateral orbital
LPL	Lipoprotein lipase
LTC	Lateral temporal cheek
MC	Middle cheek

MeC	Medial cheek
MF	Middle forehead
MRI	Magnetic resonance imaging
MSC	Mesenchymal stem cell
MTS	
NASHA	Nonanimal stabilized hyaluronic acid
NBTC	Nitroblue tetrazolium chloride
Nd:YAG	Neodymium-doped yttrium–aluminum–garnet
NL	Nasolabial
NSAID	Nonsteroidal anti-inflammatory drug
OR	
ORL	Orbital retaining ligament
PAI-1	Plasminogen activator inhibitor type 1
PAL	Power-assisted liposuction
PC/DC	Phosphatidylcholine/deoxycholate
PLLA	Poly-L-lactic acid
PMMA	Polymethylmethacrylate
PPAR	Peroxisome proliferator-activated receptor
PPLA	Polymerized polylactic acid
PRO	Patient-reported outcome
RF	Radiofrequency
SAL	Suction-assisted lipectomy or liposuction
SCS	Superficial cheek septum
SMAS	Superficial muscular aponeurotic system
SO	Supraorbital
SOOF	Suborbicularis oculi fat
TG	Triacylglyceride
TNF-α	Tumor necrosis factor alpha
UCLA	University of California Los Angeles
UCP-1	Uncoupling protein-1
WAT	White adipocyte tissue
ZM	Zygomaticus major

CHAPTER 1

Introduction

Hrak Ray Jalian[1], Alison Avram[2], and Mathew M. Avram[2]

[1] David Geffen School of Medicine, University of California Los Angeles (UCLA), CA, USA
[2] Department of Dermatology, Massachusetts General Hospital, Boston, MA

Fat is a ubiquitous component of the skin and subcutaneous tissues. In the past, many in medicine largely viewed fat as a receptacle for the passive storage of energy: a savings account of nutrients when metabolic expenditure exceeds caloric intake. However, as we pool the knowledge of fat across different specialties of medicine, we are beginning to understand the complex physiology of fat in both normal and disease states.

Dysregulation of adipose tissue, whether it be in excess in conditions such as obesity, or diminished such as in lipoatrophy, has clearly demonstrated that fat has complex metabolic, endocrine, hormonal, and immune functions (Figure 1.1). Obesity is a rising epidemic in the United States with upwards of 1 in 3 Americans being obese [1]. It has been linked to numerous chronic illnesses such as non-insulin- dependent diabetes, heart disease, liver disease, arthritis, as well as certain types of cancer [2–5].

In addition to the health consequences, these conditions often change fat distribution patterns, affecting the appearance of patients. Fat distribution has evolved to become a large component of cosmetic and procedural dermatology. In fact, as we age, cosmetic concerns regarding fat, either focal accumulation or atrophy, have become a large proportion of cosmetic consultations in physicians' offices. Currently, liposuction is one of the most common cosmetic procedures performed in the United States. Additionally, new non-invasive technologies that can successfully improve focal adiposity in the office without pain medication or sedation are becoming increasingly popular. On the other end of the spectrum, selective loss of fat, lipoatrophy, is also an emerging problem as our knowledge of facial aesthetics evolves. Focal facial volume loss can now be adequately treated

Fat removal: Invasive and non-invasive body contouring, First Edition. Edited by Mathew M. Avram.
© 2015 John Wiley & Sons, Ltd. Published 2015 by John Wiley & Sons, Ltd.

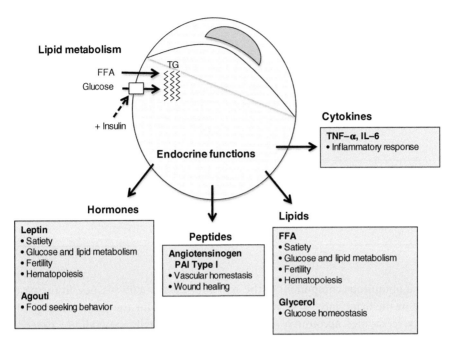

Figure 1.1 Key functions of adipocytes. Adipocytes play important roles in lipid and glucose metabolism storing them as TG. In times of energy need, these TGs are metabolized to FFA and glycerol and released into the circulation. In addition to its metabolic role, lipids, hormones, peptides, and cytokines have important endocrine roles on downstream tissue. AGT, angiotensinogen; FFA, free fatty acid; IL-6, interleukin-6; PAI-1, plasminogen activator inhibitor type 1; TG, triacylglycerol; TNF-α, tumor necrosis factor alpha.

with soft tissue augmentation and volumetric filling. Various dermal fillers have received clearance from the U.S. Food and Drug Administration (FDA) over the last decade and the number of these procedures has nearly doubled in this same time frame [6].

In order to successfully and safely perform cosmetic procedures involving the manipulation of fat, it is essential to understand the complex physiology and intricate interplay of fat as it relates to human health. Thus, it is important to gain a basic knowledge of adipogenesis, anatomy, and the physiology of fat. This chapter will serve as an abbreviated introduction to normal adipose tissue anatomy and physiology with emphasis placed on adipogenesis, the hormonal and endocrine functions of fat, and differences in adipose tissue types. This is in no way an exhaustive review, as adipose tissue is a complex organ with a multiplicity of functions, but will rather be focused on fundamental concepts that may aid in defining better treatments for conditions that are relevant to our practices.

Anatomy and physiology of adipose tissue

Fat is composed of cells known as adipocytes, the fundamental unit of fat. These cells have manifold effects on the body including energy expenditure, temperature homeostasis, and innate and adaptive immunity. Taken together, adipocytes are organized and distributed as a multi-depot organ known as adipose tissue [7]. Adipose tissue is more than just "fat" tissue. It should be thought of as a complex organ with a variety of important metabolic functions. In fact, it is composed of mature adipocytes, blood vessels, nerves, fibroblasts, and adipocyte precursor cells known as preadipocytes. Among mature adipocytes, two cytotypes can be distinguished by differences in their color and function. White adipocyte tissue (WAT) is composed of white adipocytes and macroscopically has an ivory or yellow appearance. Brown adipocyte tissue (BAT) appears brown and is composed predominantly of brown adipocytes. These two types of adipocyte tissue differ in their distribution and physiological function. Both WAT and BAT receive a vascular and nerve supply. Compared with WAT, BAT has as an abundance of mitochondria and a richer vascular tree accounts for its "brown" appearance [8]. WAT is far more abundant than BAT.

White and brown adipocytes are histologically distinct differing in size and distribution of lipid droplets and organelles [9]. White adipocytes are spherical in shape and have a single, unilocular lipid droplet occupying the cytoplasm with a relatively small eccentric nuclei rimming the periphery [10]. Brown adipocytes, in contrast, are polygonal cells with multiple smaller, "multilocular" lipid droplets, centrally placed nuclei, and a high mitochondrial content [11–13]. WAT and BAT also differ in their distribution and function. WAT is distributed in depots in two main anatomic subdivisions: intra-abdominal visceral fat and subcutaneous fat. The subcutaneous fat is further divided into superficial and deep subcutaneous tissue [14]. BAT can be found in characteristic locations in neonates including the interscapular region, neck, axilla, and around the great vessels.

White adipose tissue

The function of WAT can be largely grouped into three main categories: (i) lipid metabolism, (ii) glucose metabolism, and (iii) endocrine functions. This is a somewhat simplified break-down of the function of WAT as these functions are all intertwined and closely regulated by the same factors. Storage of energy in the form of lipids is key to the function and existence of our species. Without the ability to efficiently store energy, caloric intake from the environment would need to be continuous. Energy storage in adipose tissue allows for humans to break down nutrients in order to have a constant supply of energy between meals or even during periods of prolonged starvation. In times of energy excess, digested free fatty acids (FFA) get stored as triacylglycerides (TGs) in adipocytes [15]. TGs are high-density energy units efficiently packed within adipocytes. In times of nutritional need, TGs are broken down into FFA and glycerol, a process known as lipolysis. In turn, FFA can be oxidized through various metabolic pathways to produce adenosine triphosphate (ATP), the basic energy unit of metabolism [16]. Lipid metabolism serves as a balance between TG synthesis, fatty acid uptake, and TG hydrolysis. Multiple hormones influence the balance between catabolism versus anabolism of lipids including insulin, cortisol, testosterone, and growth hormone. Their interactions are tightly regulated and highly complex and are beyond the purview of this chapter.

WAT also has a profound impact on glucose metabolism. Adipose tissue is among few tissues that express insulin-dependent glucose transporter-4 [15]. It is an important regulator of post-prandial extracellular glucose uptake. FFA also has an effect on hepatic glucose metabolism. High levels of FFA in circulation induce hyperglycemia both by increasing hepatic gluconeogenesis and by decreasing the rate of insulin removal. This in turn potentiates peripheral hyperinsulinemia.

WAT exerts both autocrine and paracrine functions on various organs by the secretion of bioactive peptides [17, 18]. Primarily, most of the secretory factors act on other adipocytes to regulate lipid metabolism. However, several adipocytokines are now known to influence other organ systems. Leptin is an important contributor to obesity. The murine obesity phenotype was originally described in 1950 and later characterized to be a homozygous mutation in the gene encoding leptin or its receptor [19]. These mice were found to have a voracious appetite and became massively obese. Leptin influences the hypothalamus by regulating appetite. In humans, obesity is hypothesized to be associated with leptin resistance, analogous to the insulin resistance seen in diabetes. Homozygous mutations in the gene encoding leptin in humans are associated with early-onset obesity, diabetes, failure of pubertal development, and decreased growth hormone synthesis [20]. In addition to appetite regulation, leptin has a profound effect on other organ systems including the reproductive and immune systems. It has also proven to be a promising treatment for a rare form of partial lipodystrophy, resulting in normalization of glucose and triglyceride levels in these patients [21].

Other adipocytokines are known to have important functions within various organ systems. For example, the agouti-related peptide synthesized by adipocytes, controls peripheral lipid metabolism and stimulates food-seeking behavior. Angiotensinogen and plasminogen activator inhibitor type I have thrombotic and vasoconstrictive activity and play an important role in vascular health [22, 23]. With the increasing knowledge of the importance of these adipocytokines, WAT has a significant role as an endocrine organ impacting various organ systems.

Brown adipose tissue

Despite similarities in gene expression, lipid metabolism, and hormonal regulation, BAT should be viewed as an independent organ from WAT with a unique biologic role for thermoregulation [24]. BAT is characterized by the expression of uncoupling protein-1 (UCP-1) (thermogenin), a mitochondrial protein unique to brown fat [25]. UCP-1 is essential for utilization of fatty acids for the generation of heat [25].

Thermogenesis is essential in order to maintain body temperature in response to cold exposure. This so-called non-shivering thermogenesis is important for cold acclimation, fever, and arousal from hibernation [24]. UCP-1 is upregulated during episodes of cold exposure, including in the immediate postnatal period in which a neonate is forced to rapidly acclimate from physiological temperatures to ambient room temperature. In fact, newborns use 50% of caloric intake for non-shivering thermogenesis in BAT [26, 27]. Thermogenesis in BAT is controlled by the hypothalamus through the sympathetic nervous system [28, 29]. Cold exposure results in both the hyperplastic and hypertrophic development of BAT, increased mitochondrial density, and UCP-1 expression [24, 27, 29]. Increased UCP-1 expression, in turn, results in oxidative phosphorylation of fatty acids in the mitochondrial wall and the generation of heat. This intricate interplay allows attenuation of a highly responsive, internal furnace capable of acclimating to external cold stimuli.

Despite the well-characterized role of BAT in newborns, its role in adults is less well defined. Traditional view posited adult humans to be devoid of functional brown fat. This was initially supported by the observation that UCP-1 mRNA expression is lost soon after birth with subsequent loss of the protein [30]. However, with the advent of more sensitive assays, there is compelling evidence that adults continue to express markers of BAT. Low levels of UCP-1 mRNA within islands of WAT is observed in adult humans [31–34]. In fact, 1 in 200 adipocytes in WAT are actually brown adipocytes [34]. Functional studies have found that these adipocytes are responsive to normal brown adipocyte stimuli *in vitro*. Despite these findings, initial findings of functional role for BAT in adults remained elusive [24].

Recent exciting evidence has shown the presence of physiologically functional BAT in adults. One study identified thermoactive BAT in both lean and overweight men under cold exposure, but not during thermoneutral conditions [35]. Other investigators have found defined regions of functionally active BAT in adults [36]. Factors that influenced the amount of BAT included age, body mass index, sex, outdoor temperature, and beta-blocker use. Moreover, women were more likely to have BAT, and a higher density of BAT when present.

With this new paradigm shift showing the presence of physiologically significant BAT, some have postulated a relationship between BAT and obesity. Expression of UCP-1 in BAT is significantly lower in morbidly obese subjects when compared to controls [34]. Decreased BAT is observed in obese or overweight men when compared to lean cohorts. One study, found an inverse proportion between body mass index and amount of BAT, especially in older individuals. With these findings in mind, some have postulated that active BAT may preferentially oxidize lipids for the dissipation of heat rather than store them in WAT [24, 37].

Adipogenesis: from stem cell to fat cell

The prevailing view on the development of obesity centers around the concept of adipocyte hypertrophy – an increase in the size of the cell, but no increase in number. Recent evidence now supports the additional role of adipocyte hyperplasia – an increase in the number of mature adipocytes. Human adipogenesis begins in embryos and continues into the early neonatal period [38, 39]. Adipocyte development is essential as it enables neonates to cope more efficiently with intervals between food intake [40]. We now know that humans retain the ability to recruit mature adipocytes from stem cells throughout the life span in response to nutritional needs.

Mature adipocytes are derived from precursor cells known as the preadipocyte. In humans, a predetermined number of preadipocytes are programmed at an early point of embryonic development. The preadipocytes are derived from mesenchymal stem cells (MSCs) of mesoderm origin that have the potential to become adipose tissue, smooth muscle, bone, or cartilage. There is now convincing evidence of continual adipogenesis *in vivo*. Tritiated thymidine, commonly used in cell proliferation assays as a marker for cell division, has been detected in rats fed a high caloric diet suggesting adipocyte differentiation in response to a high caloric intake [41] (Figure 1.2).

In vivo studies of adipogenesis are limited for several reasons. Fat is unique as an organ system in that it exists in unevenly distributed, non-contiguous pockets throughout the body, each with its own unique molecular milieu [42]. For this reason, *in vitro* models using preadipocyte cells lines or primary preadipocytes have largely been utilized to determine the cascade of adipogenesis. The validity of these experimental models is supported by the observation that mature adipocytes derived from clonal preadipocytes *in vitro* have the same similarity in appearance and response to hormonal stimulus of adipose tissue [43]. Further, preadipocytes develop into mature adipocytes when injected into mice [44].

A complex process drives adipocyte development. Essentially this can be broken down into a two-step sequence of events: (i) recruitment and proliferation of preadipocytes and (ii) differentiation to mature adipocytes. In the first stage, there is an increased number of cells, followed by differentiation marked by a change in morphology and function of the cell. Numerous regulatory signals are involved in the complex cascade. Transition from proliferation to differentiation in cell culture involves expression of collagen VI and disappearance

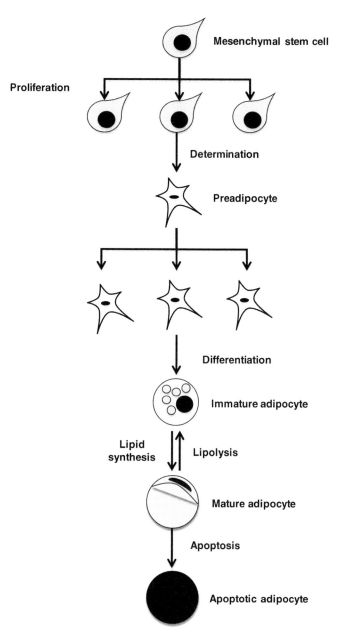

Figure 1.2 Adipocyte differentiation and proliferation. Two proliferative phases take place during adipogenesis. The first proceeds determination with replication of mesenchymal stem cells. The second occurs after determination with replication of the preadipocytes. During differentiation, stellate shaped preadipocytes become round and accumulate lipid and subsequently acquire mature adipocyte phenotype. Depending on the metabolic demands and physiologic influence, mature adipocytes can undergo apoptosis, or lose lipid, a process called lipolysis.

of inhibitory proteins. The required first step in adipocyte differentiation is growth arrest [17, 45, 46]. *In vitro* models require addition of proliferative and proadipogenic signals for induction of differentiation [47]. After induction, these preadipocytes divide and reach another growth arrest phase that is required for terminal differentiation. The most prominent of the adipogenic transcription factors are the peroxisome proliferator-activated receptors (PPARs) and the CCAAT/enhanced-binding proteins (C/EBPs). It is at this stage that the levels of these two transcription factors begin to increase. This rise is important for the preadipocyte to commit to differentiation. As levels continue to increase, downstream proteins involved in glucose and lipid metabolism increase 10- to 100-fold [17]. Synthesis of adipocyte-secreted products is a marker of late adipocyte differentiation, and establishes the organ as an important endocrine regulator of homeostasis.

As we know that adipogenesis and fat accumulation can happen over one's lifetime, it is widely accepted that adipocyte loss can also occur during this time frame [48]. Weight loss studies demonstrate a reduction in the volume and number of mature adipocytes [49, 50]. Two mechanisms are hypothesized to be responsible for this phenomenon: programmed cell death, known as apoptosis, or dedifferentiation, the process by which mature cells revert to less committed precursor cells [51–53]. Evidence for apoptosis is supported by demonstration of both a mitochondrial dependent pathway and a cell surface death signal mediated pathway *in vitro*. These pathways in turn activate a cascade of proteases, resulting in cleavage of genetic material, DNA fragmentation, and eventual phagocytosis [54]. Other tissue culture studies have revealed that adipocytes from obese persons demonstrate a relative resistant to dedifferentiation, highlighting the propensity of adipocytes to preserve their differentiated lipid-laden states [55].

Despite evidence for adipogenesis, apoptosis, and dedifferentiation, the precise number of adipocytes is tightly regulated. There is an approximate turnover of about 10% of fat cells annually [56].

Summary

As the physical and psychosocial impact of fat-related disorders grow, our knowledge of adipose tissue as an organ has been forced to keep pace. Although far from understanding the nuances of adipose tissue and its complex, far reaching physiological functions, our current comprehension paints a picture of an organ system capable of adapting to a multitude of different physiological conditions. We now understand that adipocytes are capable of both enlarging and dividing in times of metabolic excess or during cold exposure. Conversely, adipocytes can also undergo apoptosis or dedifferentiation under certain physiological conditions such as during times of weight loss.

The expanding autocrine and paracrine functions of adipose tissue solidify its role as a potent endocrine organ. Through adipocytokine signals, fat is able to influence numerous physiological functions including glucose metabolism, androgen synthesis, vascular tone, immunity, as well as other important roles. The gradation of the local hormonal milieu in each pocket of adipose tissue speaks to the intricate nature and sensitivity of adipose tissue in regards to its autocrine function.

Better experimental techniques including the use of MSCs, *ex vivo* regeneration of tissue on bioengineered scaffolds, and isolation of preadipocytes will continue to expand our understanding of the behavior of this complex organ. This increased knowledge may lead to better, targeted therapeutics aimed at addressing the underlying causes of fat-related disorders.

References

1 *Overweight and obesity.* Available from: http://www.cdc.gov/obesity/data/adult.html [cited 1 December 2011].

2 Manson, J.E. & Bassuk, S.S. (2003) Obesity in the United States: a fresh look at its high toll. *The Journal of the American Medical Association*, **289** (**2**), 229–230.

3 Matarasso, A., Kim, R.W. & Kral, J.G. (1998) The impact of liposuction on body fat. *Plastic and Reconstructive Surgery*, **102** (**5**), 1686–1689.

4 Montague, C.T. & O'Rahilly, S. (2000) The perils of portliness: causes and consequences of visceral adiposity. *Diabetes*, **49** (**6**), 883–888.

5 Stallone, D.D. (1994) The influence of obesity and its treatment on the immune system. *Nutrition Reviews*, **52** (**2 Pt 1**), 37–50.

6 *2011 Plastic surgery procedural statistics.* Available from: http://www.plasticsurgery.org/news-and-resources/2011-statistics-.html [cited 1 December 2011].

7 Cinti, S. (2002) Adipocyte differentiation and transdifferentiation: plasticity of the adipose organ. *Journal of Endocrinological Investigation*, **25** (**10**), 823–835.

8 Cinti, S. (2005) The adipose organ. *Prostaglandins, Leukotrienes, and Essential Fatty Acids*, **73** (**1**), 9–15.

9 Fawcett, D. (1952) A comparison of the histological organization and cytochemical reactions of brown and white adipose tissues. *Journal of Morphology*, **90**, 363–405.

10 Napolitano, L. (1963) The differentiation of white adipose cells. An electron microscope study. *Journal of Cell Biology*, **18**, 663–679.

11 Afzelius, B.A. (1970) Brown adipose tissues: its gross anatomy, histology, and cytology. In: Lindberg, O. (ed), *Brown Adipose Tissue*. Elsevier, Amsterdam, pp. 1–31.

12 Geloen, A. *et al.* (1990) In vivo differentiation of brown adipocytes in adult mice: an electron microscopic study. *The American Journal of Anatomy*, **188** (**4**), 366–372.

13 Napolitano, L. & Fawcett, D. (1958) The fine structure of brown adipose tissue in the newborn mouse and rat. *Journal of Biophysical and Biochemical Cytology*, **4** (**6**), 685–692.

14 Smith, S.R. *et al.* (2001) Contributions of total body fat, abdominal subcutaneous adipose tissue compartments, and visceral adipose tissue to the metabolic complications of obesity. *Metabolism*, **50** (**4**), 425–435.

15 Marks, D.B. (1996) *Basic Medical Biochemistry: a Clinical Approach.* Lippincott Williams & Williams, Philadelphia.

16 Fukuchi, K. *et al.* (2003) Visualization of interscapular brown adipose tissue using (99m)Tc-tetrofosmin in pediatric patients. *Journal of Nuclear Medicine*, **44** (**10**), 1582–1585.

17 Gregoire, F.M., Smas, C.M. & Sul, H.S. (1998) Understanding adipocyte differentiation. *Physiological Reviews*, **78** (**3**), 783–809.

18 Kim, S. & Moustaid-Moussa, N. (2000) Secretory, endocrine and autocrine/paracrine function of the adipocyte. *Journal of Nutrition*, **130** (**12**), 3110S–3115S.

19 Friedman, J.M. *et al.* (1991) Molecular mapping of the mouse ob mutation. *Genomics*, **11** (**4**), 1054–1062.

20 Clement, K. *et al.* (1998) A mutation in the human leptin receptor gene causes obesity and pituitary dysfunction. *Nature*, **392** (**6674**), 398–401.

21 Guettier, J.M. *et al.* (2008) Leptin therapy for partial lipodystrophy linked to a PPAR-gamma mutation. *Clinical Endocrinology*, **68** (**4**), 547–554.

22 Panahloo, A. & Yudkin, J.S. (1996) Diminished fibrinolysis in diabetes mellitus and its implication for diabetic vascular disease. *Coronary Artery Disease*, **7** (**10**), 723–731.

23 Tsikouris, J.P., Suarez, J.A. & Meyerrose, G.E. (2002) Plasminogen activator inhibitor-1: physiologic role, regulation, and the influence of common pharmacologic agents. *Journal of Clinical Pharmacology*, **42** (**11**), 1187–1199.

24 Cannon, B. & Nedergaard, J. (2004) Brown adipose tissue: function and physiological significance. *Physiological Reviews*, **84** (**1**), 277–359.

25 Cinti, S. *et al.* (1997) Immunohistochemical localization of leptin and uncoupling protein in white and brown adipose tissue. *Endocrinology*, **138** (**2**), 797–804.

26 Hey, E.N. (1969) The relation between environmental temperature and oxygen consumption in the new-born baby. *Journal of Physiology*, **200** (**3**), 589–603.

27 Himms-Hagen, J. (2001) Does brown adipose tissue (BAT) have a role in the physiology or treatment of human obesity? *Reviews in Endocrine & Metabolic Disorders*, **2** (**4**), 395–401.

28 Lafontan, M. & Berlan, M. (1993) Fat cell adrenergic receptors and the control of white and brown fat cell function. *Journal of Lipid Research*, **34** (**7**), 1057–1091.

29 Lowell, B.B. & Spiegelman, B.M. (2000) Towards a molecular understanding of adaptive thermogenesis. *Nature*, **404** (**6778**), 652–660.

30 Clarke, L. *et al.* (1997) Adipose tissue development during early postnatal life in ewe-reared lambs. *Experimental Physiology*, **82** (**6**), 1015–1027.

31 Champigny, O. & Ricquier, D. (1996) Evidence from in vitro differentiating cells that adrenoceptor agonists can increase uncoupling protein mRNA level in adipocytes of adult humans: an RT-PCR study. *Journal of Lipid Research*, **37** (**9**), 1907–1914.

32 Garruti, G. & Ricquier, D. (1992) Analysis of uncoupling protein and its mRNA in adipose tissue deposits of adult humans. *International Journal of Obesity and Related Metabolic Disorders*, **16** (**5**), 383–390.

33 Krief, S. *et al.* (1993) Tissue distribution of beta 3-adrenergic receptor mRNA in man. *Journal of Clinical Investigation*, **91** (**1**), 344–349.

34 Oberkofler, H. *et al.* (1997) Uncoupling protein gene: quantification of expression levels in adipose tissues of obese and non-obese humans. *Journal of Lipid Research*, **38** (**10**), 2125–2133.

35 van Marken Lichtenbelt, W.D. *et al.* (2009) Cold-activated brown adipose tissue in healthy men. *New England Journal of Medicine*, **360** (**15**), 1500–1508.

36 Cypess, A.M. *et al.* (2009) Identification and importance of brown adipose tissue in adult humans. *New England Journal of Medicine*, **360** (**15**), 1509–1517.

37 Lin, S.C. & Li, P. (2004) CIDE-A, a novel link between brown adipose tissue and obesity. *Trends in Molecular Medicine*, **10** (**9**), 434–439.

38 Burdi, A.R. *et al.* (1985) Adipose tissue growth patterns during human gestation: a histometric comparison of buccal and gluteal fat depots. *International Journal of Obesity*, **9** (**4**), 247–256.

39 Poissonnet, C.M., LaVelle, M. & Burdi, A.R. (1988) Growth and development of adipose tissue. *Journal of Pediatrics*, **113** (**1 Pt 1**), 1–9.

40 MacDougald, O.A. & Lane, M.D. (1995) Transcriptional regulation of gene expression during adipocyte differentiation. *Annual Review of Biochemistry*, **64**, 345–373.

41 Miller, W.H. Jr.,, Faust, I.M. & Hirsch, J. (1984) Demonstration of de novo production of adipocytes in adult rats by biochemical and radioautographic techniques. *Journal of Lipid Research*, **25** (**4**), 336–347.

42 Adams, M. *et al.* (1997) Activators of peroxisome proliferator-activated receptor gamma have depot-specific effects on human preadipocyte differentiation. *Journal of Clinical Investigation*, **100** (**12**), 3149–3153.

43 Rubin, C.S. *et al.* (1978) Development of hormone receptors and hormonal responsiveness in vitro. Insulin receptors and insulin sensitivity in the preadipocyte and adipocyte forms of 3T3-L1 cells. *Journal of Biological Chemistry*, **253** (**20**), 7570–7578.

44 Green, H. & Kehinde, O. (1979) Formation of normally differentiated subcutaneous fat pads by an established preadipose cell line. *Journal of Cellular Physiology*, **101** (**1**), 169–171.

45 Amri, E.Z. *et al.* (1986) Coupling of growth arrest and expression of early markers during adipose conversion of preadipocyte cell lines. *Biochemical and Biophysical Research Communications*, **137** (**2**), 903–910.

46 Smas, C.M. & Sul, H.S. (1995) Control of adipocyte differentiation. *Biochemical Journal*, **309** (**Pt 3**), 697–710.

47 Ntambi, J.M. & Young-Cheul, K. (2000) Adipocyte differentiation and gene expression. *Journal of Nutrition*, **130** (**12**), 3122S–3126S.

48 Ailhaud, G. *et al.* (1991) Growth and differentiation of regional adipose tissue: molecular and hormonal mechanisms. *International Journal of Obesity*, **15** (**Suppl. 2**), 87–90.

49 Miller, W.H. Jr., *et al.* (1983) Effects of severe long-term food deprivation and refeeding on adipose tissue cells in the rat. *American Journal of Physiology*, **245** (**1**), E74–E80.

50 Zhou, Y.T. *et al.* (1999) Reversing adipocyte differentiation: implications for treatment of obesity. *Proceedings of the National Academy of Sciences of the United States of America*, **96** (**5**), 2391–2395.

51 Sugihara, H. *et al.* (1986) Primary cultures of unilocular fat cells: characteristics of growth in vitro and changes in differentiation properties. *Differentiation*, **31** (**1**), 42–49.

52 Van, R.L., Bayliss, C.E. & Roncari, D.A. (1976) Cytological and enzymological characterization of adult human adipocyte precursors in culture. *Journal of Clinical Investigation*, **58** (**3**), 699–704.

53 Van, R.L. & Roncari, D.A. (1978) Complete differentiation of adipocyte precursors. A culture system for studying the cellular nature of adipose tissue. *Cell and Tissue Research*, **195** (**2**), 317–329.

54 Gupta, S. (2001) Molecular steps of death receptor and mitochondrial pathways of apoptosis. *Life Sciences*, **69** (**25–26**), 2957–2964.

55 Cheng, A.Y., Deitel, M. & Roncari, D.A. (1993) Relative resistance of adipocytes from massively obese persons to dedifferentiation. *Obesity Surgery*, **3** (**4**), 340–345.

56 Arner, P. *et al.* (2011) Dynamics of human adipose lipid turnover in health and metabolic disease. *Nature*, **478** (**7367**), 110–113.

CHAPTER 2

Facial fat: anatomy and implications for rejuvenation

Hrak Ray Jalian and Rebecca Fitzgerald

David Geffen School of Medicine, University of California Los Angeles (UCLA), Los Angeles, CA, USA

KEY POINTS

- Aging is a dynamic process involving characteristic changes to the skin, adipose tissue, and craniofacial skeleton.

- Facial adipose tissue exists in discrete, reproducible independent anatomical subunits referred to as fat pads.

- Loss of volume within these fat pads contributes to change in facial topography and is evidenced by "downstream" markers, such as the nasolabial fold.

- Fat pads age independently from each other and variably between individuals.

- Soft tissue augmentation with variable agents, in a targeted approach, can achieve natural restoration of youth.

Introduction

As our understanding of the dynamics of facial aging evolves, a complex paradigm involving structural changes in multiple tissue layers is emerging. What we once predominantly attributed to fragmentation of dermal collagen and mere gravitational influence on the skin and soft tissue has now morphed into a multifaceted collection of changes within the craniofacial scaffolding

Fat removal: Invasive and non-invasive body contouring, First Edition. Edited by Mathew M. Avram.
© 2015 John Wiley & Sons, Ltd. Published 2015 by John Wiley & Sons, Ltd.

and its overlying soft tissue envelope. Fat compartments play a key role in these changes.

Advances in anatomic understanding are the basis on which both surgical and nonsurgical rejuvenation techniques are designed, advanced, and refined. Rhytidectomy, for example, since its inception in the early 20th century, has evolved from simple skin excision to subcutaneous, sub-SMAS (superficial muscular aponeurotic system), deep plane, and composite dissection. Each advancement paralleled an increased understanding of the anatomy of facial structures and is a testament to the importance of detailed anatomic knowledge as the fulcrum driving improved techniques.

The last decade has shown a strong and steady movement toward non-surgical "minimally invasive" techniques with injectables and lasers. Future advancements in facial rejuvenation using these techniques will also be driven by the progress in our understanding of facial anatomy. Without regard for facial anatomy, cosmetic treatments will produce incomplete and unnatural results.

In 2007, a landmark study from Rohrich and Pessa at the University of Texas Southwestern Medical Center revolutionized our understanding of facial fat anatomy by showing that facial fat is highly compartmentalized [1]. Studies to elucidate our understanding of this facial fat anatomy have progressed rapidly since that time and are currently in a state of perpetual evolution and refinement. The value of this work lies in its implications for treatment. A more sophisticated understanding of facial fat anatomy will influence the techniques used for facial rejuvenation by furthering our ability to address site-specific corrections to achieve specific results. The goal of this chapter is to review and outline this emerging literature on facial fat anatomy and will follow a brief summary of recent literature on other structural tissue changes with age. A few clinical examples of treatment utilizing these concepts will be included for illustration.

Aging changes in multiple structural tissues

Skin

During the last decade, substantial progress has been made toward understanding the underlying mechanisms of skin aging. A major feature of aged skin is fragmentation of the dermal collagen matrix. Collagen fragmentation is responsible for loss of structural integrity and impairment of fibroblast function in senescent skin [2]. Fragmentation results from actions of specific enzymes, matrix metalloproteinases, that is observed in both intrinsic and extrinsic aging (although extrinsic aging from ultraviolet light accounts for the majority). Fibroblasts that produce and organize the collagen matrix cannot attach to fragmented collagen and they subsequently collapse. The collapsed fibroblasts produce low levels of collagen, and high levels of collagen-degrading enzymes.

Once a critical amount of collagen has been lost, this imbalance advances the aging process, in a self-perpetuating, never ending deleterious cycle. The production of new collagen demonstrated by electron microscopy after the injection of hyaluronic acid is felt likely to be due to a mechanical stretch effect, serving to rebalance collagen production and degradation, and thereby slowing its loss [3].

Muscle
The changes to the facial muscles with aging are likely multifactorial. Traditional theory was that muscles had increased laxity overtime. Recent studies suggest that the muscles of facial animation react to shifts in facial volume by increasing their resting tone. Clinically, this may have an impact on the depth at which we choose to place our fillers. If increased volume could decrease facial muscle tone, then there may be an advantage to deeper placement of facial fillers [4, 5].

Bone
Craniofacial bony remodeling is increasingly being recognized as an important contributor to the facial aging process. The landmark 2008 study by Shaw and Kahn [6–8] demonstrated statistically significant changes in the glabellar, orbital, maxillary, and pyriform angles of the facial skeleton. A recently published retrospective review of computed tomography scans of 100 patients consecutively imaged at Duke University Medical Center (including 50 men and 50 women from two age groups) found similar changes [9]. Sharabi *et al.* [10] and Mendelson *et al.* [11] have published excellent literature reviews on this topic.

Fat
As noted earlier, recent anatomic studies of the face have led to an increased understanding of the anatomy of the subcutaneous fat. For centuries, it was believed that facial fat on the face existed as one confluent mass, which eventually gets weighed down by gravity, creating sagging skin. Aesthetic facial rejuvenation therefore traditionally focused on surgical procedures, based on a paradigm of removing "excess" tissue and lifting tissues against gravity. The central role of volume loss and deflation in the aging face, rather than ptosis alone, has been compellingly illustrated by Lambros in a longitudinal photographic analysis of more than 100 patients spanning an average period of 25 years [12]. The study matched old photographs brought in by the patients with current photographs taken to match lighting and position, which were then animated using computer graphics software. These animations revealed that many facial landmarks were stable over time, eloquently demonstrating that volume loss visually mimics gravitational descent. While these animations also illustrated a somewhat predictable variability in the pace of aging between individuals, some astute observers noted a variable pace of aging within different

areas of individual faces over time, challenging the long-held assumption that the face ages as one homogeneous object and perhaps prompting some of the early studies revealing the compartmentalization of fat.

As mentioned earlier, Rohrich and Pessa's 2007 study was the first observation that superficial facial fat is organized in distinct, reproducible anatomic units. Using fresh cadavers, methylene blue dye was injected into distinct points, and cadavers were later dissected to observe dye migration. These investigators found reproducible migration and sequestration of dye, suggesting that superficial facial fat exists in independent subunits. In this initial study, distinct superficial fat compartments were described in the forehead, periorbital region, and cheek [1], some of which are illustrated in Figure 2.1.

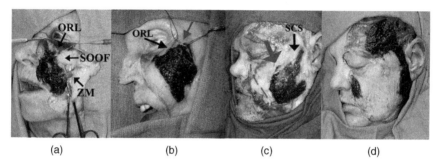

(a)   (b)   (c)   (d)

Figure 2.1 (a–d) Superficial fat compartments of the face. Methylene blue injection of facial fat pads. Nasolabial, medial cheek, middle cheek, and the large temporal lateral cheek fat compartments. Abbreviations: ORL, orbital retaining ligament; SOOF, suborbicularis oculi fat; ZM, zygomatic major muscle; SCS, superficial cheek septum. (Adapted from Rohrich & Pessa, 2007 [11]. Reproduced with permission of Lippincott Williams & Wilkins.)

Subsequent work not only validated the consistent, reproducible nature of these fat compartments, but also confirmed the presence of distinct septal barriers. Histologic evaluation of the borders of the fat compartments demonstrated a fibrous condensation of connective tissue, which forms the diffusion barrier for the dye, and separates adjacent fat compartments. These septal barriers that originated from underlying fascia, were found to be distinct from the SMAS, and inserted into the dermis [13].

There are important functional implications that come from this anatomic observation. The presence of these septal barriers forms a three-dimensional network enveloping the fat pads. This system provides scaffolding, forming a "retaining system" for the face. With these compartments so intimately intertwined, it is no surprise that volume or position change of one compartment has an effect on adjacent subunits. It is this retaining ligament system that determines the shape and location of each compartment. Moreover, in addition to their structural support of the fat pads, these retaining ligaments prevent migration of the overlying skin, a finding that is clearly evident on clinical examination. Additionally, they represent relative zones of vascularity, as evidenced by the clinical observation of alternating zones of vascularity and avascularity encountered commonly by surgeons during surgical dissection while performing facelifts. Indeed, the perforator blood supply is carried to the skin via these fibrous septations [14].

This anatomy has some important clinical implications. First, the paradigm of individual compartments with individual blood supply implies not only structural autonomy but also independent evolution with age. This echoes what we know about fat distribution through the body – despite its structural similarity, fat in different areas – is physiologically distinct. Second, because these compartments form a three-dimensional interlocking mass, volume change or migration of one pad, may cause shearing and subsequent effects on adjacent pads, affecting their spatial relationship. This, of course, makes sense intuitively and has important clinical implications regarding placement of soft tissue fillers.

The presence of reproducible fat compartments superficial to the musculature led investigators to explore and characterize the presence of fat compartments deep to the musculature. It is a well-accepted anatomic truth that fat exists both above and below facial musculature, likely to allow for the glide plane necessary for contraction. Using similar methodology visualizing dye sequestration, the deep medial cheek fat compartment was visualized [15]. This compartment, deep to the SMAS, was again an independent compartment with distinct, reproducible boundaries.

Further work revealed additional anatomic midfacial fat compartments. Dye injection studies revealed two additional compartments deep to the orbicularis oculi muscle termed the medial and lateral suborbicularis oculi fat (SOOF). These compartments, along with the deep medial cheek fat pad, form a contiguous layer of deep fat along the superior anterior maxilla and the orbital rim. Augmentation of each of these deep compartments has different effects, again underscoring the concept of site-specific augmentation.

Observations of these superficial and deep facial fat compartments prompted these researchers to posit the following: (i) changes in anterior projection and subsequent facial contour are predominantly related to volume changes of deep facial compartments (although changes in superficial fat compartments also affect contour) and (ii) folds, in contrast, manifest at transition points between superficial fat compartments of variable thickness.

The idea that deflation and volumetric change in the deep compartments lead to changes in contour and facial topography has important clinical significance. For example, the role for the medial cheek compartment is twofold. The deep medial cheek compartment is responsible not only for the anterior projection of the cheek, but also for the structural support of the overlying superficial compartments. When volume is lost in this deep compartment, the overlying skin and soft tissue envelope appear to be in excess and this manifests clinically as a more prominent nasolabial fold. This finding prompted these researchers to introduce the concept of "pseudoptosis," implying that the "ptotic" nasolabial fold is in part due to loss of anterior projection from underlying deep volume, rather than loss of volume in the area directly under the fold. Site-specific volumization of this underlying deep medial cheek fat compartment immediately manifests as increased anterior projection of the superficial fat compartments of the medial cheek, with subsequent improvement in the nasolabial fold, as well as improvement in the nasojugal fold, or "tear trough". This is well illustrated in an image of a cadaver before and after saline injected into the deep medial cheek compartment on the left side of the face (Figure 2.2). A clinical example of a similar result done using filler in a patient in this area is illustrated in Figure 2.3. In an analogous sense, the deep medial and lateral SOOF compartments of the cheek contribute to mid and lateral cheek projection. Note that the collapsed empty lateral SOOF compartment becomes more clearly visible at the superior lateral border of the "filled" deep medial cheek fat pad in the "after" image and that the absence of volume here seems to truncate the superior lateral aspect of

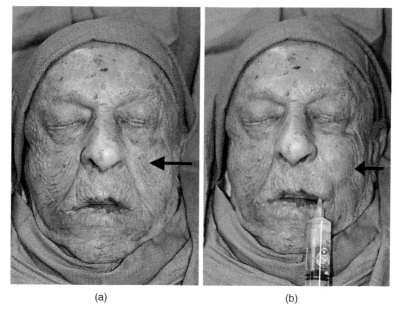

(a)   (b)

Figure 2.2 Deep medial cheek fat compartment augmentation, before (a) and after (b) saline injection. Saline injected specifically into the deep medial cheek fat compartment restores anterior projection, diminishes the nasolabial fold, and effaces the nasojugal trough. The fascial boundaries of the deep medial cheek compartment determine and define its shape. This means that filler placed specifically into this fat compartment will reflect this shape and have a natural appearance. (Source: Rohrich, 2007 [1] & Reece et al., 2008 [19]. Reproduced with permission of Lippincott Williams & Wilkins.)

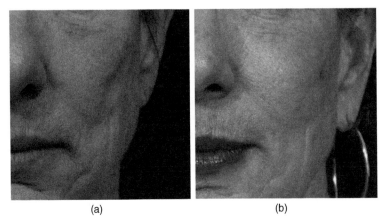

(a)   (b)

Figure 2.3 Deep medial cheek fat compartment augmentation. Clinical example of treatment in the same area as the cadaver pictured in the previous figure. Before (a) and after (b) filler injection into this anatomic compartment in this 60-year-old female patient. Again, treatment of this one area leads to effacement of the nasolabial fold and improvement in undereye hollowing. (Source: Photograph courtesy of Rebecca Fitzgerald, MD, Los Angeles, CA.)

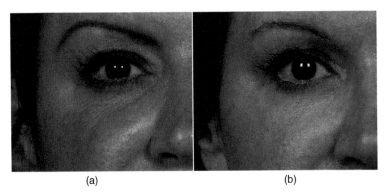

(a)   (b)

Figure 2.4 Medial and lateral SOOF augmentation. At first glance, the patient's issue seems to be a prominent nasolabial fold, but knowledge of the specific fat compartments facilitates recognition of the relatively empty medial and lateral SOOF compartments. (a) Before and (b) after filler injection into these anatomic compartments in this 38-year-old female patient. Note improvement in lateral projection and convexity of zygomatic arch. (Source: Rohrich & Pessa, 2007, 2008 [11, 12]. Reproduced with permission of Lippincott Williams & Wilkins.)

the cheek. Augmentation of this area with fillers in a patient in order to restore this area to its youthful fullness is illustrated in Figure 2.4.

These anatomic studies initiated the delineation of the structural anatomy of the facial fat compartments. More recently, advances in visualization of these facial fat pads was made possible by Gierloff *et al.* [16, 17] utilizing a novel radiopaque dye in combination with computed tomography scans providing images such as that seen in Figure 2.5. The clinical implications of

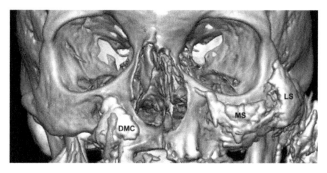

Figure 2.5 Computed tomography scan with radiopaque dye image of the deep midfacial fat compartments. The deep medial cheek fat is composed of a medial part (DMC) and a lateral part (not shown). The medial part extends medially almost to the lateral incisor tooth. Augmentation of the deep medial cheek fat will consequently elevate and efface the nasolabial fold. The suborbicularis oculi fat is composed of a medial part (MS) and a lateral part (LS). With aging, an inferior migration of these compartments occurs, as well as an inferior volume shift within the compartments. (Source: Gierloff *et al.* [16]; with permission.)

this technical achievement are twofold. First, the observer is no longer confined to standardized views in the anatomy laboratory, but is able to visualize these anatomic compartments in 3D, opening the door to new observations. For example, new observations using this technique revealed that the deep medial cheek fat pad exists as both a medial and a lateral compartment and that

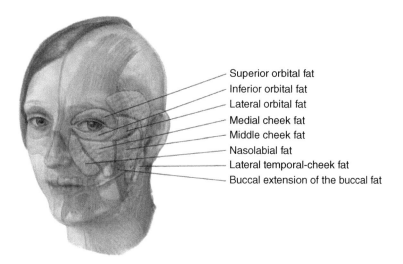

Figure 2.6 Stylistic drawing of the anatomic relationships of the facial fat compartments. The midfacial fat is arranged in two and paranasally in three independent anatomic layers. The superficial layer (yellow) is composed of the nasolabial fat, the medial cheek fat, the middle cheek fat, the lateral temporal cheek compartment, and three orbital compartments. (Source: Gierloff *et al.* [16]; reproduced with permission.)

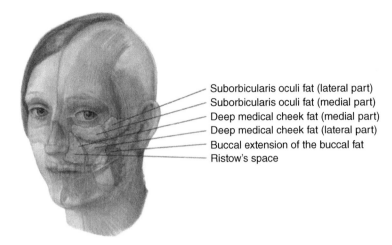

Suborbicularis oculi fat (lateral part)
Suborbicularis oculi fat (medial part)
Deep medical cheek fat (medial part)
Deep medical cheek fat (lateral part)
Buccal extension of the buccal fat
Ristow's space

Figure 2.7 Stylistic drawing of the anatomic relationships of deep midfacial fat compartments. It is composed of the suborbicularis oculi fat (medial and lateral parts) and the deep medial cheek fat (medial and lateral parts). Three layers of distinct fat compartments are found laterally to the pyriform aperture, where a deep compartment (blue) is located posterior to the medial part of the deep medial cheek fat. The buccal extension of the buccal fat pad extends from the paramaxillary space to the subcutaneous plane. (Source: Gierloff *et al.* [16]; with permission.)

an independent "buccal extention" of the buccal fat pad exists in the cheek. Findings were otherwise consistent with those described in the original dye sequestration studies done by Rohrich and Pessa, confirming their findings. Stylistic drawings depicting the superficial and deep fat compartments described in Geirloff's study are shown in Figures 2.6 and 2.7. The second clinical implication of this technique is its ability to enable subcutaneous fat compartments to now be simultaneously identified and measured. The ability of this technique to facilitate volumetric measurements of the fat compartments led these researchers to speculate that it is not only volume loss that defines the aging fat pad, but also volume redistribution within individual compartments over time [16]. This is illustrated in Figure 2.5.

Summary

Basic concepts and principles of facial anatomy enable us to systematically visualize and analyze the human face. The anatomic studies described above provide an introduction and overview of the structural anatomy of the facial fat compartments. Through this extensive, groundbreaking work we now know that facial fat is highly compartmentalized, separated by septal barriers made of fibrous membranes. The presence of these septal barriers forms a three-dimensional network enveloping the fat pads. This system provides scaffolding, forming a "retaining system" for the face. As these compartments are structurally and physiologically distinct, they may age independently. Volumetric changes in individual compartments may manifest clinically in a myriad of predictable changes (i.e., "pseudoptosis" of the nasolabial fold and development of the infraorbital "V-shaped" deformity secondary to loss of volume in the medial aspect of the deep medial cheek compartment). This anatomy has a significant clinical impact on both facial aging and facial revolumizing. By understanding the anatomy and observing the individual changes present, site-specific augmentation can better predict and target a specific area allowing for a natural appearing outcome.

In a recent comprehensive and beautifully illustrated text, Rohrich and Pessa present detailed dissections that "show" rather than "tell" this story, illustrating that the surface of the face is a roadmap for the underlying anatomy. This detailed work is an invaluable contribution to all students of anatomy, whatever their level of expertise, and is highly recommended [18].

Conclusions/future directions

Although anatomic structures show a remarkable consistency between individuals, it is the difference in the shapes of facial structures and their relationship to one another that determine the unique and distinct appearance of each individual. Therefore, as we all know, there is no "cookie cutter" ideal for all patients. Approaching the face from the standpoint of volume loss adds another paradigm to facial rejuvenation. Instead of simply excising and lifting issues, the volume paradigm invokes the concept of "filling" the lost volume of the face. Knowledge of the anatomy of the facial fat compartments allow for thoughtful analysis of the anatomy of each particular patient at a particular point in time and may help to predict and target of "site-specific" treatment in order to achieve natural appearing results and maximize both patient and physician satisfaction.

New technologies that allow us to recognize and assess three-dimensional changes will further our knowledge and techniques. Additionally, advances that make quantitative as well as qualitative evaluation possible, such as that described above will further our ability to objectively measure anatomic changes with age.

References

1 Rohrich, R.J. & Pessa, J.E. (2007) The fat compartments of the face: anatomy and clinical implications for cosmetic surgery. *Plastic and Reconstructive Surgery*, **119** (**7**), 2219–2227; discussion 2228–2231.

2 Fisher, G.J., Varani, J. & Voorhees, J.J. (2008) Looking older: fibroblast collapse and therapeutic implications. *Archives of Dermatology*, **144** (**5**), 666–672.

3 Wang, F. *et al.* (2007) In vivo stimulation of de novo collagen production caused by cross-linked hyaluronic acid dermal filler injections in photodamaged human skin. *Archives of Dermatology*, **143** (**2**), 155–163.

4 Pessa, J.E. *et al.* (1998) Relative maxillary retrusion as a natural consequence of aging: combining skeletal and soft-tissue changes into an integrated model of midfacial aging. *Plastic and Reconstructive Surgery*, **102** (**1**), 205–212.

5 Le Louarn, C., Buthiau, D. & Buis, J. (2007) Structural aging: the facial recurve concept. *Aesthetic Plastic Surgery*, **31** (**3**), 213–218.

6 Kahn, D.M. & Shaw, R.B. Jr. (2008) Aging of the bony orbit: a three-dimensional computed tomographic study. *Aesthetic Surgery Journal*, **28** (**3**), 258–264.

7 Shaw, R.B. Jr. & Kahn, D.M. (2007) Aging of the midface bony elements: a three-dimensional computed tomographic study. *Plastic and Reconstructive Surgery*, **119** (**2**), 675–681; discussion 682–683.

8 Shaw, R.B. Jr. *et al.* (2010) Aging of the mandible and its aesthetic implications. *Plastic and Reconstructive Surgery*, **125** (**1**), 332–342.

9 Richard, M.J. *et al.* (2009) Analysis of the anatomic changes of the aging facial skeleton using computer-assisted tomography. *Ophthalmic Plastic and Reconstructive Surgery*, **25** (**5**), 382–386.

10 Sharabi, S.E. *et al.* (2010) Mechanotransduction: the missing link in the facial aging puzzle? *Aesthetic Plastic Surgery*, **34** (**5**), 603–611.

11 Mendelson, B. & Wong, C. (2012) Changes in the facial skeleton with aging: implications and clinical applications in facial rejuvenation. *Aesthetic Plastic Surgery*, **36**, 753–760.

12 Lambros, V. (2007) Observations on periorbital and midface aging. *Plastic and Reconstructive Surgery*, **120** (**5**), 1367–1376; discussion 1377.

13 Rohrich, R.J. & Pessa, J.E. (2008) The retaining system of the face: histologic evaluation of the septal boundaries of the subcutaneous fat compartments. *Plastic and Reconstructive Surgery*, **121** (**5**), 1804–1809.

14 Schaverien, M.V., Pessa, J.E. & Rohrich, R.J. (2009) Vascularized membranes determine the anatomical boundaries of the subcutaneous fat compartments. *Plastic and Reconstructive Surgery*, **123** (**2**), 695–700.

15 Rohrich, R., Pessa, J. & Ristow, B. (2008) The youthful cheek and the deep medial fat compartment. *Plastic and Reconstructive Surgery*, **121**, 2107–2112.

16 Gierloff, M. *et al.* (2012) Aging changes of the midfacial fat compartments: a computed tomographic study. *Plastic and Reconstructive Surgery*, **129** (**1**), 263–273.

17 Gierloff, M. *et al.* (2012) The subcutaneous fat compartments in relation to aesthetically important facial folds and rhytides. *Journal of Plastic, Reconstructive & Aesthetic Surgery*, **65** (**10**), 1292–1297.

18 Pessa, J.E. & Rohrich, R.J. (2012) *Facial Topography: Clinical Anatomy of the Face*. Quality Medical Publishing, St. Louis, MO.

19 Reece, EM *et al.* (2008) *Plast Reconstr Surg.*, **121** (**4**), 1414–20.

CHAPTER 3

Histology and pathology of subcutaneous tissue

Selim M. Nasser[1] and Zeina S. Tannous[2]

[1] *Lebanese American University, Beirut, Lebanon*
[2] *Massachusetts General Hospital, Harvard Medical School, MA, USA*

This chapter gives an overview of the histology of normal subcutaneous tissue and also briefly discusses the tumors and inflammatory processes affecting subcutaneous fat.

White adipose tissue

Histology

White adipose tissue is widely present throughout the body and organized into collections called "depots." Most of these depots are subcutaneous, intra-abdominal or visceral. It is mainly subcutaneous fat that comes to attention for cosmetic concerns.

Adipose tissue is composed of fat cells, also called adipocytes or lipocytes. They are large spherical cells measuring 80–120 μm in diameter, containing a characteristic large lipid vacuole that occupies most of the cytoplasm and displaces an oval or flattened nucleus to the periphery (Figure 3.1a,b). In routine hematoxylin–eosin sections, these cells appear empty because of dissolution of fat during tissue processing. In the subcutis, the adipocytes are organized into lobules that are separated by septae of connective tissue. These fibrous septae are in continuity with the overlying dermis and contain arterial, venous, and

---

Fat removal: Invasive and non-invasive body contouring, First Edition. Edited by Mathew M. Avram.
© 2015 John Wiley & Sons, Ltd. Published 2015 by John Wiley & Sons, Ltd.

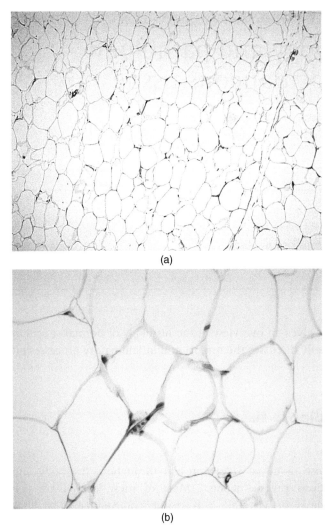
(a)

(b)

Figure 3.1 (a,b) Adipocytes with peripheral nuclei: In routine sections, the cytoplasm appears empty because of dissolution of fat during tissue processing (H&E, 200×).

lymphatic vessels and nerves (Figure 3.2). Each lobule is supplied by an arteriole that subdivides into branches and capillaries supplying microlobules and surrounding individual adipocytes. Postcapillary venules drain in septal veins. There are no capillary connections between adjacent microlobules [1].

Physiology
Fat has long been regarded as a tissue that stores excess energy and insulates the body, but our understanding of its functions has been expanding. Adipose tissue plays a major role in lipid metabolism. Fat cells store excess fatty acids

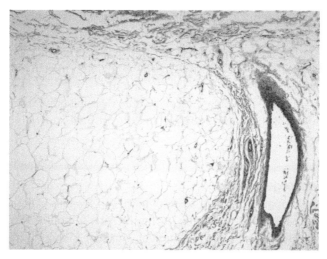

Figure 3.2 Subcutaneous fat lobule. Note the fibrous septum with blood vessels on the right hand side (H&E, 100×).

from nutrients in the form of triacylglycerol (triglyceride) to constitute energy stores for the body [2]. When needed, triacylglycerol is hydrolyzed into glycerol and free fatty acids that are released into the circulation. Fatty acids are then oxidized in other tissues to provide the main source of energy: adenosine triphosphate (ATP) [2]. Triacylglycerol can provide enormous amounts of energy, thus allowing the body to maintain all its functions between meals and, if needed, during long fasting periods [3]. Adipocyte functions can be altered by insulin, cortisol, catecholamines, growth hormone, testosterone, and cytokines [4].

Adipocytes can affect glucose metabolism by regulating the insulin-dependent glucose transporter 4, a peptide that plays a role in the transport of glucose from the circulation into cells [2]. Also, when adipocytes release free fatty acids, the effect on the liver is to promote hyperglycemia [5]. In addition, free fatty acids decrease the sensitivity of skeletal muscle to insulin and contribute to insulin resistance.

Adipose tissue can affect other tissues via endocrine, paracrine, and autocrine signals [6]. Most factors secreted from adipose tissue act in an autocrine/paracrine manner to regulate adipocyte metabolism. In addition, through the capillary network that surrounds them, adipocytes communicate with the blood stream and produce many factors and hormones. Some of these secreted factors are called adipocytokines due to similar features with cytokines [7]. Leptin is an adipocytokine with numerous paracrine and endocrine functions. It has an effect on appetite as well as on insulin regulation. It can affect steroid production as well as hematopoietic and immune development [8]. Other adipocytokines include tumor necrosis factor-α (TNF-α) and adiponectin [9, 10].

Fat cells can also produce factors that have important roles within the vascular system. They produce proinflammatory agents that may have a role in the development of cardiovascular diseases [11–13]. They also produce proteins with thrombotic and vasoconstrictor activity such as angiotensinogen and plasminogen activator inhibitor [14–16].

Additional functions of adipose tissue include roles in body contour, stem cell regeneration, and "identification" of infective organisms by providing them with specific fatty acids [17].

Growth and regulation

Adipose tissue formation can first be recognized at 14 weeks of gestation and is closely associated with angiogenesis. During the first 6 months of life, fat cells increase in size but are not much in number. During childhood, the number of fat cells increase in parallel with the body until puberty, when fat cells increase significantly both in size and in number to reach the numbers seen in adulthood [18]. The difference in fat content and distribution between men and women begins in childhood and is enhanced during puberty [18].

The number of fat cells in adults may remain stable or can increase or decrease according to diet and other factors. Infact, in contrast to most other tissues, adipose tissue volumes can increase or decrease widely [19]. It can constitute less than 10% of the weight of lean adults or increase to more than 70% of the weight of obese persons. [20–23]. Adipose tissue growth is first accomplished through an increase in the size of adipocytes (also called hypertrophy) until a "critical cell size" is reached. It is then followed by an increase in the number of adipocytes (also called hyperplasia) [22, 24, 25]. Hyperplasia involves precursor cells' (preadipocytes) replication/differentiation program [26–33]. Modest weight gain results usually from adipocyte hypertrophy while severe obesity is associated with both hypertrophy and hyperplasia of fat cells [19].

During weight loss, there is a reduction in both adipocyte number and volume [22]. Reduction in food intake is associated mainly with reduction in adipocyte volume [34], but significant weight loss includes reduction in adipocyte number which is accomplished through apoptosis and adipocyte dedifferentiation. Apoptosis is the ability of adipocytes to undergo regulated cell death. It has been observed *in vitro* and it plays a role in pathologic conditions associated with weight loss, such as malignancy and protease inhibitor-associated lipodystrophy in HIV disease [35–37]. Adipocyte dedifferentiation is a process in which mature adipocytes revert morphologically and biochemically to a less differentiated precursor cell type [32, 38–41].

Adipose tissue mass is determined by the net balance between energy consumption and energy intake. The latter is determined by dietary intake, while the former is determined by homeostatic metabolic processes such as physical activity and thermogenesis [42–44]. Basal metabolic rate is modulated by body temperature, thyroid status, pregnancy, lactation, gender, and age [19]. More particularly, the increase or decrease in the number of fat cells is controlled by several factors. Those include regulators that promote increased adipocytes, such as insulin, glucocorticoid, and polyunsaturated fatty acids and regulators that decrease the number of fat cells, such as leptin, retinoids, and TNF-α [19, 45]. Interestingly, it appears that these regulators may not affect the increase or decrease of adipocytes of different regions in the body equally. This may provide some explanation to the unequal distribution of fat depot in the subcutis in some individuals [46, 47].

Brown adipose tissue

Histology

Brown adipose tissue is the adipose tissue that appears brown and contains adipocytes called "brown adipocytes", which are different from white adipocytes. They are smaller (20–40 mm) and polygonal with centrally located nuclei. They are characterized by the presence of numerous large mitochondria within the cytoplasm. In contrast to white adipocytes, where lipids are organized into a single vacuole, lipids in brown adipocytes form multiple smaller "multilocular" droplets [48–50], conferring a foamy or bubbly appearance to these cells (Figure 3.3). Compared with its white counterpart, brown adipose tissue contains a much richer vascular supply, which together with the abundant mitochondria confer a brown coloration to this tissue.

Brown adipose tissue can be identified at the 20th week of pregnancy, later than its white counterpart [2]. Its development continues until shortly after

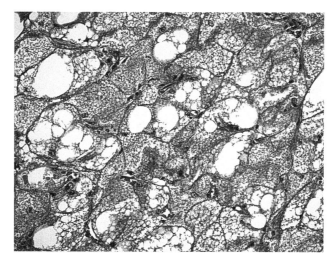

Figure 3.3 Brown adipose tissue. Note the numerous smaller fat droplets inside the adipocyte cytoplasm (H&E, 200×).

birth. In newborn and young children, it can be present in several areas, more particularly in the interscapular region and surrounding large blood vessels, in the neck, the axillae, thoracic cavity, and abdomen [51–53]. In humans, brown adipose tissue is progressively transformed and replaced by white adipose tissue [54, 55] so that in adults conspicuous depots of brown fat are not identified. However, this belief has been recently revised by studies that have demonstrated that some white adipocytes can transform, under certain conditions, into brown adipocytes [54, 56, 57]. Moreover, studies that detect the presence of uncoupling protein-1 (UCP-1), a protein specific of brown adipocytes, have demonstrated the existence of scattered brown adipocytes within collections of white adipose tissue [58–62].

Physiology

Similar to white adipose tissue, brown adipose tissue synthesizes and hydrolyzes lipids and secretes hormones such as leptin [63]. However, it is characterized by a specific mitochondrial protein, the UCP-1 (or thermogenin). This protein is present exclusively in brown adipose tissue and its main function is to uncouple the oxidation of fatty acid from the production of ATP resulting in the transformation of fatty acid energy into heat [64–66]. Therefore, UCP-1 confers brown adipose tissue, its major function in thermogenesis in the human neonates as well as in rodents and hibernators. As the brown adipose tissue appears to transform fatty acids into heat, it may have a potential role in the protection from obesity [67–69].

Tumors of fat

Lipoma is the most common soft tissue tumor in adults. Conventional lipoma is usually a well-circumscribed mass of mature adipose tissue composed of adipocytes that vary widely in size (Figure 3.4). In addition to conventional lipoma, several other variants are described such as angiolipoma, mixoid lipoma, fibrolipoma, and spindle cell lipoma. Lipomas are most commonly located in the subcutis. They are best treated with surgical excision.

Liposarcoma is a rare malignant tumor of adipose tissue usually located in the deep soft tissues and retroperitoneum. Several types of liposarcoma are described. Some types are associated with indolent behavior, other types follow an aggressive course.

Lipoblastoma is a rare benign tumor composed of immature (fetal-like) adipose tissue occurring usually before the age of 3 years.

Hibernoma is a rare and benign tumor composed of mature brown adipose tissue [70].

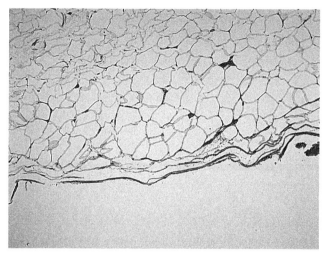

Figure 3.4 Lipoma: A tumor composed of mature adipocytes surrounded by a thin fibrous capsule (H&E, 200×).

Panniculitis

The hallmark of panniculitis is inflammation of subcutaneous fat. It can be divided into septal and lobular pannicultis [71, 72].

Septal panniculitis
Septal panniculitis is the inflammation of the connective tissue septae with some spillover to the adjacent fat (Figure 3.5). In chronic septal panniculitis, the septae might be widened with some reduction in the size of the fat lobules.

Conditions with septal panniculitis include erythema nodosum (EN), necrobiosis lipoidica, and scleroderma. The most common cause of septal panniculitis is *erythema nodosum*. EN presents as painful erythematous nodules usually on the lower legs, with or without associated systemic symptoms. It can be idiopathic, infection-induced, drug-induced, pregnancy-associated, or can be a manifestation of a systemic disorder such as sarcoidosis, lymphoproliferative disorders, connective tissue diseases, and inflammatory bowel disease.

Lobular panniculitis
In lobular panniculitis, the inflammatory infiltrate involves the entire lobule with some septal involvement (Figure 3.6). Causes of lobular panniculitis include erythema induratum, subcutaneous fat necrosis of the newborn, sclerema neonatorum, poststeroid panniculitis, pancreatic panniculitis, lupus panniculitis, infection associated panniculitis, and traumatic panniculitis.

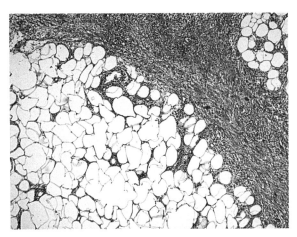

Figure 3.5 Septal pannicultis. A fat lobule is surrounded by a fibrous septum with chronic inflammation. Note that there is some spillover of inflammatory cells to the fat lobule (H&E 2×, 100×).

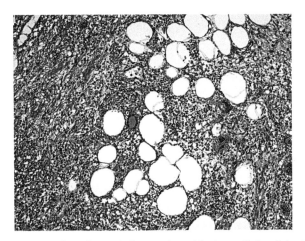

Figure 3.6 Lobular pannicultis: Chronic inflammation with giant cells involving intalobular adipose tissue (H&E, 200×).

Erythema induratum presents as red nodules or plaques on posterior legs that can ulcerate and drain. It is usually associated with tuberculosis, but also associated with other infections, drugs, or can be idiopathic. The histology is characterized by the presence of lobular panniculitis, vasculitis, mixed inflammatory cell infiltrate, and granuloma formation.

Subcutaneous fat necrosis of the newborn, sclerema neonatorum, and poststeroid panniculitis occur in infants and children. They present as hardening of the skin or erythematous subcutaneous nodules and are characterized by the formation of crystals within the adipocytes because of higher ratio of saturated/unsaturated fatty acids in young fat, unlike adult fat. Histology reveals lobular panniculitis with needle-shaped clefts in fat cells. Sclerema neonatorum shows less or no inflammation.

Pancreatic panniculitis is associated with pancreatitis or pancreatic cancer. It presents with erythematous subcutaneous nodules with systemic symptoms. The histology is characterized by the presence of lobular panniculitis with ghost-like necrotic adipocytes and deposition of basophilic material.

Lupus panniculitis presents as subcutaneous nodules that can be painful. It is often associated with cutaneous or systemic lupus and can sometimes precede other lupus manifestations. The histology is characterized by the presence of lobular lymphohistiocytic panniculitis with hyaline necrosis and paraseptal lymphoid follicles. It is often associated with lupus changes in the epidermis and dermis.

Infection associated panniculitis can be caused by multiple infections including fungi, bacteria, and mycobacteria. The histology is nonspecific and manifests as lobular pannicultis with numerous neutrophils, granulomas, necrosis, and hemorrhage. Special stains are needed to identify the organism.

Traumatic panniculitis presents as firm subcutaneous nodules at the sites of injury. It can be caused by physical or chemical injury.

Physical injury causing traumatic panniculitis:

Physical injury can be in the form of cold exposure or blunt trauma. Other physical insults include excessive heat or electrical injury.

Cold panniculitis occurs after exposure to severe cold. Infants and children are more susceptible to cold injury because of their higher ratio of saturated to unsaturated fat that raises the crystallization temperature of the young fat leading to cold panniculitis. It can occur in children on the cheeks and chin after eating iced popsicles (pospicle panniculitis). It can also occur in adults such as on the thighs of women after riding horses while wearing tight pants (equestrian panniculitis). Histopathology of cold panniculitis reveals deep perivascular lymphohistiocytic infiltrate and lobular panniculitis with a mixed inflammatory cell infiltrate predominantly adjacent to the dermosubcutaneous junction. The infiltrate consists of lymphocytes, foamy macrophages, neutrophils, and occasional eosinophils with adipocyte necrosis, rupture, and microcyst formation. Unlike subcutaneous fat necrosis of the newborn, needle-shaped clefts are not seen in cold panniculitis. This type of panniculitis has been of particular interest in the field of cosmetic surgery as it served as the inspiration for cryolipolysis treatment for the noninvasive removal of fat.

Blunt trauma-induced panniculitis occur predominantly on the arms or hands and is frequently associated with ecchymosis. Histopathology reveals organizing hematoma with hemosiderin deposition

Other forms of panniculitis:

Injected chemicals can also cause traumatic panniculitis. *Factitial panniculitis* results from self-injection of a variety of substances in the fat such as milk, and urine and feces by psychiatrically ill patients. *Sclerosing lipogranuloma* (paraffinoma) of the male genitalia or female breasts results from self-injection of lipid materials such as mineral oil (paraffin) or other oils in the fat. Chemical-induced panniculitis can be produced by multiple *injectable therapeutic agents* such as interleukin-2, interferon alpha, meperidine, pentazocine, povidone, morphine, and phytonadione (vitamin K). Panniculitis can also be produced from injection of foreign materials into the skin for cosmetic purposes such as lipid materials, mesotherapy injections, or silicone that may contain impurities such as olive oil or castor oil.

The injection of various agents into the fat produces lobular panniculitis with a variety of histologic findings. Acute lesions show focal fat necrosis with neutrophilic infiltration and hemorrhage (Figure 3.7). Older lesions show lymphohistiocytic infiltrates with macrophages and fibrosis. Identification of the exogenous material using polarized light or performing lipid stains of frozen sections is essential for diagnosis. Injection of oily materials such as in sclerosing lipogranuloma will produce granulomatous lobular panniculitis and characteristic "swiss cheese appearance". There are multiple round or oval vacuoles and fat cysts with foamy macrophages and foreign body giant cells with surrounding fibrosis. These conditions are challenging to treat.

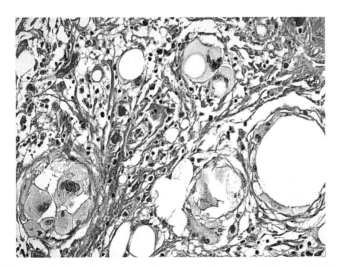

Figure 3.7 Fat necrosis: The adipocytes are disrupted and surrounded by lymphohistiocytic inflammatory infiltrate including numerous giant cells (H&E, 400×).

Panniculitis induced by cosmetic procedures

Many cosmetic modalities have been recently developed to eliminate excess fat deposits. These new technologies usually induce a lobular panniculitis that leads to fat necrosis and subsequently to fat loss in certain areas of the body where body sculpting is desired. Cryolipolysis induces cold panniculitis, a subtype of traumatic lobular panniculitis induced by cold exposure [73]. Laser-assisted liposuction induces traumatic panniculitis that is induced by heat generated from laser light directly in contact with the fat. The laser-induced heat liquefies fat and makes it easily suctioned with the liposuction cannula [74]. The 1210 nm laser can induce selective photothermolysis of adipose tissue while sparing the overlying epidermis and the dermis [75, 76]. Injection adipolysis or adipolytic therapy usually utilizes injectable detergents such as sodium deoxycholate or phosphatidylcholine to ablate or destroy adipose tissue by solubilizing the adipocyte cell membrane [77].

References

1 Requena, L. (2007) Normal subcutaneous fat, necrosis of adipocytes and classification of the panniculitides. *Seminars in Cutaneous Medicine and Surgery*, **26**, 66–70.

2 Avram, A., Avram, M. & James, W. (2005) Subcutaneous fat in normal and diseased states: 2. Anatomy and physiology of white and brown adipose tissue. *Journal of the American Academy of Dermatology*, **53**, 671–683.

3 Van Dijk, G. (2001) The role of leptin in the regulation of energy balance and adiposity. *Journal of Neuroendocrinology*, **13**, 913–921.

4 Ramsay, T.G. (1996) Fat cells. *Endocrinology and Metabolism Clinics of North America*, **25**, 847–870.

5 Wajchenberg, B.L. (2000) Subcutaneous and visceral adipose tissue: their relation to the metabolic syndrome. *Endocrine Reviews*, **21**, 697–738.

6 Kim, S. & Moustaid-Moussa, N. (2000) Secretory, endocrine and autocrine/paracrine function of the adipocyte. *Journal of Nutrition*, **130**, 3110S–3115S.

7 Trayhurn, P. & Beattie, J.H. (2001) Physiological role of adipose tissue: white adipose tissue as an endocrine and secretory organ. *Proceedings of the Nutrition Society*, **60**, 329–339.

8 Zhang, Y., Proenca, R., Maffei, M., Barone, M., Leopold, L. & Friedman, J.M. (1994) Positional cloning of the mouse obese gene and its human homologue. *Nature*, **372**, 425–432.

9 Kern, P.A., Saghizadeh, M., Ong, J.M., Bosch, R.J., Deem, R. & Simsolo, R.B. (1995) The expression of tumor necrosis factor-α in human adipose tissue. Regulation by obesity, weight loss, and relationship to lipoprotein lipase. *Journal of Clinical Investigation*, **95**, 2111–2119.

10 Hotamisligil, G.S., Shargill, N.S. & Spiegelman, B.M. (1993) Adipose expression of tumor necrosis factor-a: direct role in obesity-linked insulin resistance. *Science*, **259**, 87–91.

11 Ridker, P.M., Rifai, N., Rose, L., Buring, J.E. & Cook, N.R. (2002) Comparison of C-reactive protein and low-density lipoprotein cholesterol levels in the prediction of first cardiovascular events. *New England Journal of Medicine*, **347**, 1557–1565.

12 Ridker, P.M., Rifai, N., Stampfer, M.J. & Hennekens, C.H. (2000) Plasma concentration of interleukin-6 and the risk of future myocardial infarction among apparently healthy men. *Circulation*, **101**, 1767–1772.

13 Yudkin, J.S., Kumari, M., Humphries, S.E. & Mohamed-Ali, V. (2000) Inflammation, obesity, stress and coronary heart disease: is interleukin-6 the link? *Atherosclerosis*, **148**, 209–214.

14 Engeli, S., Negrel, R. & Sharma, A. (2000) Physiology and pathophysiology of the adipose tissue renin–angiotensin system. *Hypertension*, **35**, 1270–1277.

15 Tsikouris, J.P., Suarez, J.A. & Meyerrose, G.E. (2002) Plasminogen activator inhibitor-1: physiologic role, regulation, and the influence of common pharmacologic agents. *Journal of Clinical Pharmacology*, **42**, 1187–1199.

16 Panahloo, A. & Yudkin, J.S. (1996) Diminished fibrinolysis in diabetes mellitus and its implication for diabetic vascular disease. *Coronary Artery Disease*, **7**, 723–731.

17 Klein, J. *et al.* (2007) What are subcutaneous adipocytes really good for … ? *Experimental Dermatology*, **16**, 45–70.

18 Poissonnet, C.M., LaVelle, M. & Burdi, A.R. (1988) Growth and development of adipose tissue. *Journal of Pediatrics*, **113**, 1–9.

19 Avram, A., Avram, M. & James, W. (2005) *Journal of the American Academy of Dermatology*, **53**, 663–670.

20 Knittle, J.L., Timmers, K. & Ginsberg-Felner, F. (1979) The growth of adipose tissue in children and adolescents: cross sectional and longitudinal studies of adipose cell number and size. *Journal of Clinical Investigation*, **63**, 239–246.

21 Sjostrom, L. & William-Olsson, T. (1981) Prospective studies on adipose tissue development in man. *International Journal of Obesity*, **5**, 597–604.

22 Prins, J.B. & O'Rahilly, S. (1997) Regulation of adipose cell number in man. *Clinical Science*, **92**, 3–11.

23 Hausman, D.B., DiGirolamo, M., Bartness, T.J., Hausman, G.J. & Martin, R.J. (2001) The biology of white adipocyte proliferation. *Obesity Reviews*, **2**, 239–254.

24 Bjorntorp, P. (1991) Adipose tissue distribution and function. *International Journal of Obesity and Related Metabolic Disorders*, **15**, 67–81.

25 Faust, I.M. & Miller, H.M. Jr. (1983) Hyperplastic growth of adipose tissue in obesity. In: Angel, A., Hollenberg, C.H. & Roncari, D.A.K. (eds), *The Adipocyte and Obesity: Cellular and Molecular Mechanisms*. Raven Press, New York, pp. 41–51.

26 Ng, C.W., Poznanski, W.J., Borowiecki, M. & Reimer, G. (1971) Differences in growth in vitro of adipose cells from normal and obese patients. *Nature*, **231**, 445.

27 Morrison, R.F. & Farmer, S.R. (2000) Hormonal signaling and transcriptional control of adipocyte differentiation. *Journal of Nutrition*, **130** (**Suppl.**), S3116–S3121.

28 Rosen, E.D. & Spiegelman, B.M. (2000) Molecular regulation of adipogenesis. *Annual Review of Cell and Developmental Biology*, **16**, 145–171.

29 Spiegelman, B.M. & Flier, J.S. (1996) Adipogenesis and obesity: rounding out the big picture. *Cell*, **87**, 377–389.

30 Ntambi, J.M. & Kim, Y.-C. (2000) Adipocyte differentiation and gene expression. *Journal of Nutrition*, **130** (**Suppl.**), S3122–S3126.

31 Gregoire, F.M., Smas, C.M. & Sul, H.S. (1998) Understanding adipocyte differentiation. *Physiological Reviews*, **78**, 783–809.

32 Van, R.L. & Roncari, D.A. (1978) Complete differentiation of adipocyte precursors: a culture system for studying the cellular nature of adipose tissue. *Cell and Tissue Research*, **195**, 317–329.

33 Poznanski, W.J., Waheed, I. & Van, R. (1973) Human fat cell precursors. *Laboratory Investigation*, **29**, 570–576.

34 Yang, M.U., Presta, E. & Bjorntorp, P. (1990) Refeeding after fasting in rats: effects of duration of starvation and refeeding on food efficiency in diet-induced obesity. *American Journal of Clinical Nutrition*, **51**, 970–978.

35 Domingo, P., Matias-Guiu, X., Pujol, R.M. *et al.* (1999) Subcutaneous adipocyte apoptosis in HIV-1 protease inhibitor-associated lipodystrophy. *AIDS*, **13**, 2261–2267.

36 Flier, J.S. (2000) Pushing the envelope on lipodystrophy. *Nature Genetics*, **24**, 103–104.

37 Carr, A., Samara, K., Chisholm, D.J. & Cooper, D.A. (1998) Pathogenesis of HIV-1 protease inhibitor-associated peripheral lipodystrophy, hyperlipidemia, and insulin resistance. *Lancet*, **351**, 1881–1883.

38 Fernyhough, M.E., Helterline, D.L., Vierck, J.L., Hausman, G.J., Hill, R.A. & Dodson, M.V. (2005) Dedifferentiation of mature adipocytes to form adipofibroblasts: more than just a possibility. *Adipocytes*, **1**, 17–24.

39 Sugihara, H., Yonemitsu, N., Miyabara, S. & Yun, K. (1986) Primary cultures of unilocular fat cells: characteristics of growth in vitro and changes in differentiation properties. *Differentiation*, **31**, 42–49.

40 Van, R.L.R., Bayliss, C.E. & Roncini, D.A.K. (1976) Cytological and enzymological characterization of adult human adipocyte precursors in culture. *Journal of Clinical Investigation*, **58**, 688–704.

41 Cancello, R., Pietri-Rouxel, F. & Clement, K. (2005) Spontaneous lipid accumulation in primary cultures of dedifferentiated human adipocytes. *Adipocytes*, **1**, 73–78.

42 Spiegelman, B.M. & Flier, J.S. (2001) Obesity and the regulation of energy balance. *Cell*, **104**, 531–543.

43 Barsh, G.S. & Schwartz, M.W. (2002) Genetic approaches to studying energy balance: perception and integration. *Nature Reviews Genetics*, **3**, 589–600.

44 Loftus, T.M. (1999) An adipocyte-central nervous system regulatory loop in the control of adipose homeostasis. *Seminars in Cell and Developmental Biology*, **10**, 11–18.

45 Gullicksen, P.S., Della-Fera, M.A. & Baile, C.A. (2003) Leptin-induced adipose apoptosis: implications for body weight regulation. *Apoptosis*, **8**, 327–335.

46 Papineau, D., Gagnon, A.M. & Sorisky, A. (2003) Apoptosis of human abdominal preadipocytes before and after differentiation into adipocytes in culture. *Metabolism*, **52**, 987–992.

47 Niesler, C.U., Siddle, K. & Prins, J.B. (1998) Human preadipocytes display a depot-specific susceptibility to apoptosis. *Diabetes*, **47**, 1365–1368.

48 Afzelius, B.A. (1970) Brown adipose tissue: its gross anatomy, histology and cytology. In: Lindberg, O. (ed), *Brown Adipose Tissue*. Elsevier, Amsterdam, pp. 1–31.

49 Geloen, A., Collet, A.J., Guay, G. & Bukowiecki, L.J. (1990) In vivo differentiation of brown adipocytes in adult mice: an electron microscopic study. *The American Journal of Anatomy*, **188**, 366–372.

50 Napolitano, L. & Fawcett, D. (1958) The fine structure of brown adipose tissue in the newborn mouse and rat. *Journal of Biophysical and Biochemical Cytology*, **4**, 685–690.

51 Lean, M.E. (1989) Brown adipose tissue in humans. *Proceedings of the Nutrition Society*, **48**, 243–256.

52 Okuyama, C., Ushijima, Y., Kubota, T. *et al.* (2003) 123I-Metaiodobenzylguanidine uptake in the nape of the neck of children: likely visualization of brown adipose tissue. *Journal of Nuclear Medicine*, **44**, 1421–1425.

53 Fukuchi, K., Ono, Y., Nakahata, Y., Okada, Y., Hayashida, K. & Ishida, Y. (2003) Visualization of interscapular brown adipose tissue using (99m) Tc-tetrofosmin in pediatric patients. *Journal of Nuclear Medicine*, **44**, 1582–1585.

54 Himms-Hagen, J. (2001) Does brown adipose tissue (BAT) have a role in the physiology or treatment of human obesity? *Reviews in Endocrine & Metabolic Disorders*, **2**, 395–401.

55 Penicaud, L., Cousin, B., Leloup, C., Lorsignol, A. & Casteilla, L. (2000) The autonomic nervous system, adipose tissue plasticity, and energy balance. *Nutrition*, **16**, 903–908.

56 Tiraby, C., Tavernier, G., Lefort, C. *et al.* (2003) Acquirement of brown fat cell features by human white adipocytes. *Journal of Biological Chemistry*, **278**, 33370–33376.

57 Hansen, J.B., te Riele, H. & Kristiansen, K. (2004) Novel function of the retinoblastoma protein in fat: regulation of white versus brown adipocyte differentiation. *Cell Cycle*, **6**, 774–778.

58 Champigny, O. & Ricquier, D. (1996) Evidence from in vitro differentiating cells that adrenoreceptor agonists can increase uncoupling protein mRNA levels in adipocytes of adult humans: an RT-PCR study. *Journal of Lipid Research*, **37**, 1907–1914.

59 Garruti, G. & Ricquier, D. (1992) Analysis of uncoupling protein and its mRNA in adipose tissue deposits of adult humans. *International Journal of Obesity*, **16**, 383–390.

60 Oberkofler, H., Dallinger, G., Liu, Y.M., Hell, E., Krempler, F. & Patsch, W. (1997) Uncoupling protein gene: quantification of expression levels in adipose tissues of obese and non-obese humans. *Journal of Lipid Research*, **38**, 2125–2133.

61 Krief, S., Lonnqvist, F., Raimbault, S. *et al.* (1993) Tissue distribution of b3-adrenergic receptor mRNA in man. *Journal of Clinical Investigation*, **91**, 344–349.

62 Cousin, B., Cinti, S., Morroni, M. *et al.* (1992) Occurrence of brown adipocytes in rat white adipose tissue: molecular and morphological characterization. *Journal of Cell Science*, **103**, 931–942.

63 Cinti, S., Frederich, R.C., Zingaretti, M.C., De Matteis, R., Flier, J.S. & Lowell, B.B. (1997) Immunohistochemical localisation of leptin and uncoupling protein in white and brown adipose tissue. *Endocrinology*, **138**, 797–804.

64 Klingenberg, M. & Winkler, E. (1985) The reconstituted isolated uncoupling protein is a membrane potential-driven H1 translocator. *EMBO Journal*, **4**, 3086–3092.

65 Garlid, K.D., Jaburek, M. & Jezek, P. (1998) The mechanism of proton transport mediated by mitochondrial uncoupling proteins. *FEBS Letters*, **438**, 10–14.

66 Klingenberg, M. & Huang, S.G. (1999) Structure and function of the uncoupling protein from brown adipose tissue. *Biochimica et Biophysica Acta*, **1415**, 271–296.

67 Giacobino, J.-P. (2002) Uncoupling proteins, leptin, and obesity: an updated review. *Annals of the New York Academy of Sciences*, **967**, 398–402.

68 Lowell, B.B. & Flier, J.S. (1997) Brown adipose tissue, b3-adrenergic receptors, and obesity. *Annual Review of Medicine*, **48**, 307–316.

69 Mattson, M.P. (2010) Does brown fat protect against diseases of aging? *Ageing Research Reviews*, **9 (1)**, 69–76.

70 Weiss, S. & Goldblum, J. (2007) *Enzinger and Weiss's Soft Tissue Tumors*, Fifth edn. Mosby, USA.

71 Weedon, D. (2010) *Weedon's Skin Pathology*, Third edn. Elsevier, USA.

72 Bolognia, J., Jorizzo, J. & Rapini, R. (2008) *Dermatology*, Second edn. Mosby/Elsevier, USA.

73 Zelickson, B., Egbert, B.M., Preciado, J. *et al.* (2009) Cryolipolysis for noninvasive fat cell destruction: initial results from a pig model. *Dermatologic Surgery*, **35 (10)**, 1462–1470.

74 Palm, M.D. & Goldman, M.P. (2009) Laser lipolysis: current practices. *Seminars in Cutaneous Medicine and Surgery*, **28 (4)**, 212–219.

75 Anderson, R.R., Farinelli, W., Laubach, H. *et al.* (2006) Selective photothermolysis of lipid-rich tissues: a free electron laser study. *Lasers in Surgery and Medicine*, **38 (10)**, 913–919.

76 Wanner, M., Avram, M., Gagnon, D. *et al.* (2009) Effects of non-invasive, 1,210 nm laser exposure on adipose tissue: results of a human pilot study. *Lasers in Surgery and Medicine*, **41 (6)**, 401–407.

77 Rotunda, A.M. (2009) Injectable treatments for adipose tissue: terminology, mechanism, and tissue interactions. *Lasers in Surgery and Medicine*, **41 (10)**, 714–720.

CHAPTER 4

Injectable treatments for fat and cellulite

Adam M. Rotunda*

David Geffen School of Medicine, University of California Los Angeles (UCLA), CA, USA

KEY POINTS

- This chapter reviews the history of injectable treatments for small collections of fat, with an emphasis on clarifying terminology and mechanism of action of several medications in development.

- Lipodissolve® (an injectable combination of phosphatidylcholine and sodium deoxycholate) and mesotherapy employ unregulated, compounded medications that have been associated with significant adverse events.

- An adipolytic medication based on purified, nonanimal derived sodium deoxycholate is in FDA registration trials for the reduction of submental fat.

- A lipolytic medication, a combination of a β-agonist (salmeterol xinafoate) and a steroid (fluticasone propionate), is in FDA registration trials for the reduction of abdominal fat and exophthalmos.

- There is currently no data to suggest that injectable medications for cellulite are safe or efficacious.

*Dr. Rotunda is a consultant to KYTHERA Biopharmaceuticals, Lithera, and Allergan.

Fat removal: Invasive and non-invasive body contouring, First Edition. Edited by Mathew M. Avram.
© 2015 John Wiley & Sons, Ltd. Published 2015 by John Wiley & Sons, Ltd.

Introduction

Subcutaneous injections that reduce adipose tissue have been most frequently referred to as injection lipolysis, phosphatidylcholine/deoxycholate (PC/DC), Lipodissolve®, and mesotherapy [1–5]. These terms are outdated and associated with controversial, unregulated treatments. Injectable treatments for fat dissolution in development are intended to reduce small pockets of fat, not as a tool for large surface area body contouring. Pharmaceutical grade, injectable medications that permanently or non-permanently remove small collections of fat have aptly been referred to as *adipolytic therapy* and *pharmaceutical lipoplasty*, respectively.

If current investigations lead to U.S. Food and Drug Administration (FDA) approved drugs, the procedure may very well broaden the pool of aesthetic physicians who treat fat, as well as open a new market of patients who seek minimally invasive aesthetic treatments. However, the history of fat reducing with injections is marred with controversy. It may therefore be reasonable to view new data about these therapies with a sense of caution and anticipation.

The popularity of colloquially termed "fat melting" injections can be attributed in part to the Lipodissolve marketing campaign by Fig. (formerly American Lipodissolve, St. Louis, MO) commercial treatment centers and the American Society for Aesthetic Lipodissolve (ASAL). As of this writing, however, no commercially available injectable formulations are approved anywhere worldwide for fat removal. FDA considers injectable fat reduction "unapproved drugs for unapproved uses ... ," [6] and even its illicit use persists. Notorious reports of cutaneous infections and necrosis, corporate bankruptcies, medical society warning statements, as well as state legislation banning the procedure [7–14], have contributed to the infamy of this treatment. Despite the alarm, validation of efficacy and an acceptable safety profile by recent well-controlled investigations are evidence for the increasingly exciting prospect of offering patients a nonsurgical, nondevice, and minimally invasive remedy to reduce fat.

As none of these medications are in current commercial production, this chapter does not fit neatly into the layout used in the rest of this book (patient selection, consultation, procedure, etc.). Given this constraint, however, the background and research behind an innovative line of medication may be of interest to some readers who wish to be on the "cutting" edge.

Clarification of terms and history

Lipolysis, injection lipolysis, pharmaceutical lipoplasty, adipolysis, and adipolytic therapy

The term *lipolysis* describes the hydrolysis, or degradation, of lipids into their constituent fatty acid and glycerol building blocks [15]. Lipolysis results in the

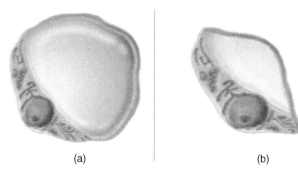

(a)   (b)

Figure 4.1 (a) Schematic representation of adipocyte at baseline. (b) Schematic representation of adipocyte lipolysis; adipocyte reduces volume following hormone sensitive lipase activation and subsequent release of glycerol and free fatty acids. (Source: Adam M. Rotunda. Reproduced with permission of Adam M. Rotunda.)

reduction of fat cell volume while preserving the cell viability (Figure 4.1). Lipolysis occurs within adipocytes and vascular lumen of muscle and fat tissue, and is regulated by hormone sensitive lipase (HSL) and lipoprotein lipase (LPL), respectively [15]. HSL is expressed in adipose tissue and is activated by cortisone and catecholamines, which are lipolytic, and inhibited by insulin, which is lipogenic. LPL is located on endothelial walls of capillaries and is responsible for serum chylomicron (from dietary lipids) and very low-density lipoprotein breakdown. Lipolysis may also be induced by medication binding to specific adrenergic receptors (α or β) located on adipocyte membranes [15–18].

A novel medication currently being developed by Lithera, Inc. (San Diego, CA) is termed "LIPO-102" and its use as an injectable fat reducer is called "pharmaceutical lipoplasty." Understandably, the company prefers this term to "injection lipolysis" although "injection lipolysis" is technically (physiologically) accurate. "Injection lipolysis" has been historically associated with Lipodissolve or PC/DC injections, which carry a tarnished past. Adding to the confusion, "injection lipolysis" should never have been used to describe treatments that incorporate the detergent, DC. Any detergent-based formulation elicits adipocyte lysis, and so it will not effectively stimulate adipocyte lipolysis, which is a process that requires a fully functioning, or viable, fat cell. Therefore, in order to more accurately describe injectable methods that employ detergents to diminish fat, the terms, "adipolysis" or "adipolytic therapy," are preferred [19].

Brief history of mesotherapy, Lipostabil®, Lipodissolve®, and the role of the compounding pharmacy

The term *mesotherapy* should not be used interchangeable with PC/DC, DC, Lipodissolve, injection lipolysis, pharmaceutical lipoplasty, or adipolytic therapy [2, 4, 5, 20]. The repeated, incorrect use of the term in the lay and medical litera-ture has inadvertently confused physicians and patients. Mesotherapy (from the

Greek mesos, "middle" and therapeia, "to treat medically") was first introduced in 1952 by French physician Pistor [21] and describes cutaneous injections of minute doses of medication. Mesotherapy has been recognized and traditionally practiced in Europe as a localized treatment in pain medicine, sports medicine, and rheumatology, but has been applied over time to cosmetic medicine for conditions such as alopecia, cellulite, photoaging, and scarring [1, 4, 5, 22, 21]. The nature of the target condition determines at what depth (epidermal, dermal, or subcutaneous) the injections (often hundreds) of extemporaneously mixed combinations of vasodilators, anti-inflammatory agents, herbs, hormones, antibiotics, enzymes, or coenzymes are placed with a syringe, injection gun, or multineedle device [1, 4, 5, 22]. Several small, yet well-designed studies have generated renewed interest in this traditional form of mesotherapy as a treatment for a number of aesthetic and medical conditions [23–26].

Lipostabil® (Sanofi-Aventis, Paris, France) "fat melting" injections were introduced onto the worldwide stage by Rittes [27], a dermatologist in São Paolo, Brazil, who reported reduction of infraorbital fat using direct, transcutaneous injection with Lipostabil. Lipostabil is manufactured and marketed for intravenous use in Europe, South American, and South Africa as a treatment for numerous fat-related disorders (i.e., hyperlipidemia, angina pectoris, diabetic angiopathy). Lipostabil consists of soy-derived PC (5%), its solvent sodium deoxycholate (2.5%), DL-α-tocopherol (vitamin E), sodium hydroxide, ethanol, and benzyl alcohol, in sterile water.

Importing Lipostabil into the United States is illegal, and there are no approved PC/DC or DC medications for which physicians can use "off-label." To meet the demand by physicians and patients, compounding pharmacies have produced formulations similar to Lipostabil; the most popular was Lipodissolve. The now defunct company, Fig. (formerly American Lipodissolve, St. Louis, MO), popularized a chain of treatment centers that used compounded medications of PC and DC based loosely on the original Lipostabil formulation. Compounded formulations generally consists of 5% PC combined with 4.2–4.75% DC [2, 3, 5] or 1–5% DC alone [2, 3, 28–31]. At times, collagenase or lipolytic agents (i.e., caffeine, isoproterenol, yohimbine) were added to purportedly [18] augment fat reduction. In the United States, these medications are legally available through compounding [2, 5], although the concentration and purity of medication formulated at a compounding pharmacy can be dubious [32]. As malpractice coverage and standards of care between state and region, physicians may be placing themselves in a precarious position by treating patients with unapproved medication.

Regulations pertaining to compounding vary by state [2, 5]. Traditional compounding involves preparing a specialized, custom drug product to fill an individual patient's prescription when an approved drug cannot meet their needs. With regard to PC/DC, it appears that most, if not all, of the compounded formulations are performed in bulk in anticipation of receiving sales in mass quantities. Interestingly, PC/DC is not being compounded for an individually identified patient, and pharmacies are compounding preestablished and unregulated formulations (i.e., they are not produced within facilities meeting cGMP (Current Good Manufacturing Practice) regulations enforced by the FDA). Local and systemic safety margins of deoxycholate using a cGMP formulation are being used in pivotal clinical studies.

Over the past decade, investigations by Dr. Rittes [33–35] and others [2, 22, 20, 36, 28, 37–39, 29, 40–42, 30, 43, 31, 44, 45] have reported that Lipostabil, compounded PC/DC, and compounded DC reduce fat on the hips, the abdomen, the back rolls (known affectionately as "love handles" in men or "bra strap fat" in women), dorsocervical region ("buffalo hump"), the neck, the jowls, and the lipomas (Figure 4.2). Two relatively recently conducted, IRB-approved

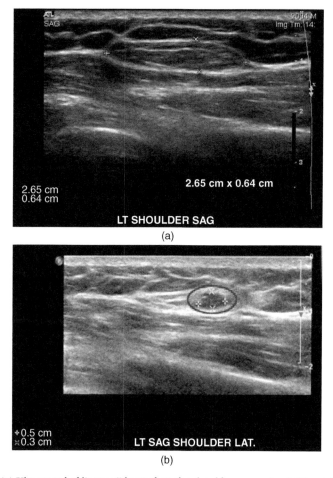

Figure 4.2 (a) Ultrasound of lipoma 7 located on the shoulder measuring $2.65\,cm \times 0.64\,cm$ before sodium deoxycholate (10 mg/mL) treatment. (b) Same lipoma measuring $0.5\,cm \times 0.3\,cm$ 4 months after second and last injection.

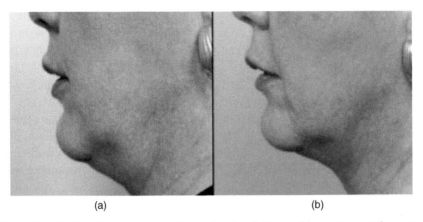

(a)   (b)

Figure 4.3 Subject profile before (a) and 2 months after (b) 5 monthly injections with 1.0 mL of compounded sodium deoxycholate (10 mg/mL) into the submental fat area.

prospective, randomized, double-blind clinical trials with compounded PC/DC and DC alone in submental fat [3] (Figure 4.3) and hips [30] and have substantiated the beneficial clinical effects of these medication observed in prior case series and retrospective studies. The indications, technique, safety profile, and so-called "standards of practice" (a paradox in light of its unregulated use) of PC/DC or Lipodissolve techniques therapy have been reviewed [2, 3, 35]. However, all of these reports utilize non-pharmaceutical grade (non-cGMP medication) DC derived from bovine sources, using anecdotal, nonstandardized techniques.

Clarifying the roles of deoxycholate and phosphatidylcholine

The PC hypothesis

The preponderance of published literature on the subject of injectable fat treatments describes treatment with PC/DC or DC alone. Basic science research, detailed below, has revealed that, invariably, a component of all these formulations was the biologic detergent, DC. It is generally accepted that all published reports describing injectable PC formulations contain DC.

Early publications [27, 43, 46] hypothesized that the lecithin-derived phospholipid, PC, was the active fat-reducing ingredient in Lipostabil. The premise was that the same mechanism responsible for reducing serum lipids by PC in intravenous Lipostabil (for which it is approved in Europe) was effective to reduce subcutaneous fat tissue. It was also conjectured [16, 46] that PC induced a cascade of intracellular signals that led to apoptosis, or that it directly lysed fat cell membranes, emulsified triglycerides, upregulated LPL, and facilitated transit of triglycerides across cell membranes. None of these theories could be supported experimentally.

Focus on DC

Deoxycholic acid (Figure 4.4) is a secondary bile acid produced by intestinal bacteria after the release of primary bile acids (i.e., cholic acid) in the liver [5]. Biologically compatible detergents such as DC have been conventionally used to improve the solubility of the major constituents of intravenous medications, such as Amphotericin B (Amphocin®, Pfizer) [5]. Sodium deoxycholate is the solvent for PC in Lipostabil, as phospholipids such as PC are essentially water insoluble [47].

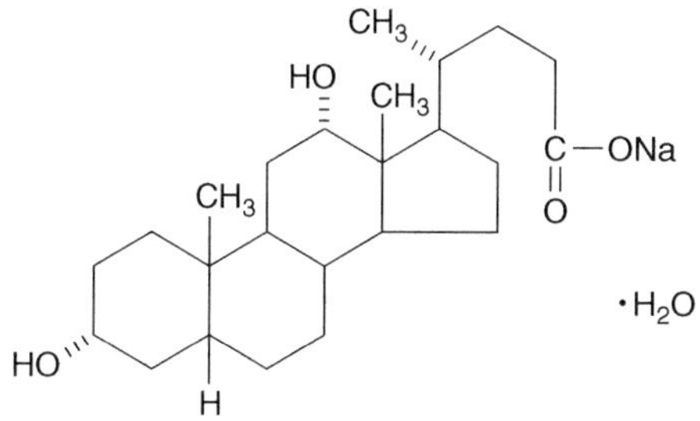

Figure 4.4 Chemical structure of sodium deoxycholate.

An unforeseen discovery [45] revealed that DC alone (without PC) produced cell death and cell lysis *in vitro* (keratinocytes) and *ex vivo* (pig adipose tissue) equal to the effects produced by the PC/DC combination (Figure 4.5). These were the first data that called into question the role of PC as the fat-reducing agent by demonstrating that the bile salt, DC, produces nonspecific cell lysis independent of PC.

The strength of the argument that DC acted as the sole active ingredient was based on a mounting evidence from independent sources. Gupta *et al.* [48] demonstrated that DC alone and PC/DC are comparably cytotoxic on cultured adipocytes, endothelial cells, fibroblasts, and skeletal muscle cells. Schuller-Petrovic *et al.* [28] extended these laboratory findings into living tissue by performing cell lysis and cell viability studies *in vivo* (rat adipose tissue) using PC/DC and isolated DC (Figure 4.6). Additional experiments have corroborated the lytic effects of DC on adipocytes *in vivo* and *in vitro* [49, 50]. This laboratory and animal data has been validated through human studies that demonstrate comparable fat-reducing effects when either DC or PC/DC are injected into lipomas [40, 31, 44], abdominal [2, 29], submental [3], and hip fat [2, 3, 29, 40, 41, 30].

Deoxycholate is an ionic detergent that disrupts the integrity of biological membrane by introducing their polar hydroxyl groups into the cell membrane's

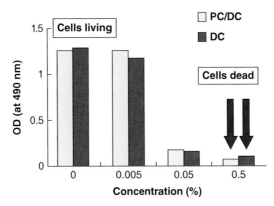

Figure 4.5 MTS cell viability assay measuring living keratinocytes exposed to phosphatidylcholine/deoxycholate (PC/DC) and deoxycholate (DC). Absorbance (OD) is directly related to cell viability. Increasing concentration of either PC/DC or DC alone produces cell death. DC alone profoundly reduces cell viability, with PC producing minimal effect. (Source: Adam M. Rotunda. Reproduced with permission of Adam M. Rotunda.)

phospholipid bilayer hydrophobic core [51]. The process involves first an "attack" of the detergent on the membrane; solubilization of membrane-associated proteins; saturation of the membrane with detergent; and finally, with increasing detergent concentration, membrane integrity breakdown, and solubilysis [51–54] (Figure 4.7).

While the role of PC as an active participant in localized fat loss had been called into question for years [16, 19, 28–30, 45, 48], the contention that PC itself could not lyse cells or reduce fat was based only on indirect evidence. Some authors contended that the inclusion of PC was historical artifact [5, 16]. There appeared to be minimal difference in experimental and clinical outcomes when PC was added to DC, and so PC itself was presumed yield minimal or no fat-reducing effects. Being water soluble, DC's effect on cells and tissue was relatively straightforward to quantify experimentally. On the other hand, it was technically difficult to evaluate PC's direct effect on cells and fat tissue because of its insolubility in the aqueous solutions used in all the prior studies. Conventional laboratory phospholipid solvents such as chloroform and ethanol are membrane toxic. This problem was not solved for years.

Duncan and colleagues [2] resolve this quandary by designing a novel method to investigate the effect of PC on adipocytes using mineral oil as its solvent, which could dissolve PC but not affect cell membranes. In this way, the isolated effect of PC on cells could be observed without the confounding lytic effects of PC's solvent. The authors incubated human-derived adipocyte stem cells from abdominal fat and induced them to maturity. Cytotoxicity assays (lactate dehydrogenase and oil red O) and lipolysis assays (glycerol and triglyceride assays) were performed on the cultured adipocytes after exposure to PC (5%)/mineral oil, DC

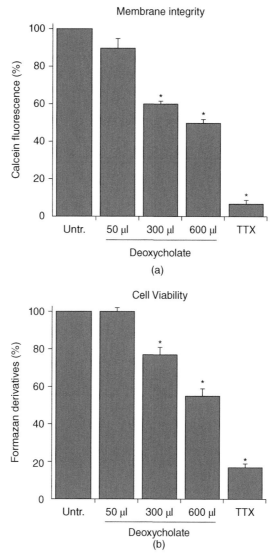

Figure 4.6 Effects of DC (2.5%) on (a) rat fat cell membrane integrity and (b) cell viability after repetitive dosing. The effects were observed after 30 days following application of DC on days 0, 7, and 28. Triton (TTX) 0.5% served as positive control. These data translate the experimental data summarized in Figure 4.5 into a living model. (Source: Medical Insight, Inc., Chicago, IL. Reproduced with permission of Medical Insight, Inc.)

(1% and 2.4%), benzyl alcohol, and isoproterenol (a β-agonist) (Table 4.1). These data are the first to experimentally confirm that PC has no adipolytic (i.e., fat cell lysing) or lipolytic (i.e., triglyceride degrading) effects.

Despite evidence that DC is the sole active ingredient, some clinicians maintain that it is safer for the patient to incorporate PC with DC. To their credit, there

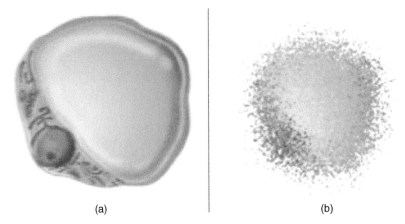

(a)   (b)

Figure 4.7 (a) Schematic representation of adipocyte at baseline. (b) Schematic representation of adipolysis; adipocyte becomes nonviable following membrane solubilysis and degradation by detergent.

Table 4.1 PC in isolation from DC neither cause adipolysis (fat cell lysis) nor lipolysis (triglyceride breakdown). These data are the first to experimentally confirm prior deductions that PC will not reduce fat without DC.

Test solution	Adipocyte cell lysis obtained with this solution
PC50/DC42	++
Deoxycholate 1%	+++
Deoxycholate 2.4%	+++
Phosphatidylcholine 5% in mineral oil	0
Isuprel 0.08% injectable	0
Local anesthetic 5%	0
Saline 0.9% (control)	0
Benzyl alcohol	0

Source: Diane Duncan. Reproduced with permission of Diane Duncan.

is evidence that relatively high concentrations (>1%) of DC alone produce profound inflammation, prolonged nodularity, and potentially, skin necrosis [2, 29, 43, 31, 45], while PC/DC combinations that use high concentrations of DC (until 4.75%) appear less likely to produce these outcomes [2, 30]. In an effort to identify what effects, if any, PC had on the lytic activity of DC, Bentow *et al.* [55] found that in the presence of PC, almost 10 times more DC was required to lyse adipocytes, and that there is a threefold reduction in the area of fat necrosis as compared to when DC was used alone (Figure 4.8). These results may be a consequence of DC and PC spontaneously forming detergent/phospholipid aggregates

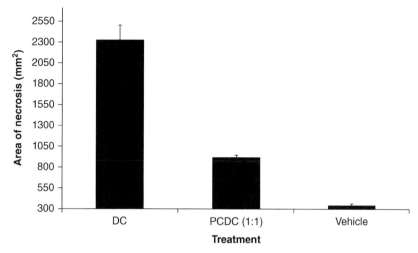

Figure 4.8 Inclusion of 0.5% PC with 0.5% DC produces a threefold reduction in fat cell death (as measured by area of necrosis *in vivo*) compared to 0.5% DC. PC inhibits the desirable fat-reducing effect of DC. (Source: Bentow *et al.* (2009) [55].)

called micelles [47, 51]; while unbound DC is capable of lysing fat tissue, it is reasonable to assume that PC/DC micelles have no or minimal lytic capacity [3, 55]. Rather than "protective," PC *inhibits* the desirable fat-reducing effects of DC.

A small, double-blind study investigating submental fat reduction demonstrated no differences in efficacy or safety of a low-concentration (1%) DC formulation compared to a PC (5%)/DC (4.75%) formulation. Low dose DC appears to be an efficacious and safe concentration for subcutaneous injection [3, 31, 44, 56].

There are no data from large-scale, rigorous (controlled, randomized, and blinded) trials to conclude any advantage of using PC with DC. As with most drugs, a safe and effective single ingredient medication is more desirable than a multi-ingredient formulation, unless the latter possesses significant advantages.

Detergents and tissue interactions

Mechanism of fat reduction and further implications on efficacy and safety

Fundamentally akin to sclerotherapy [57], subcutaneously injected DC necroses tissue as a result of its cytotoxic effects on the cellular membranes. Isolated DC causes adipocytes to lyse and release their triglyceride contents in the extracellular environment [56]. Almost immediately, inflammation and edema manifest clinically. Living and *ex vivo* animal human tissue exposed to DC, as well as

PC/DC combinations, demonstrate fat cell lysis; erythrocytes extravasation; and a mixed infiltrate consisting of polymorphonuclear leukocytes, lymphocytes, macrophages, and multinucleated giant cells; and fibrosis [2, 5, 34, 28, 29, 40, 41, 31, 45, 58, 49]. The visible gross and histological progression of events that occurs following detergent injection into a lipoma has been documented [31] (Figure 4.9). Controlled adipolysis and moderate degrees of postinflammatory

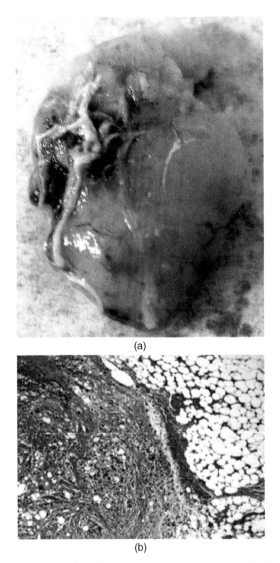

(a)

(b)

Figure 4.9 (a) Excised lipoma 2 days after injection with sodium deoxycholate (10 mg/mL) revealing a well-demarcated area of necrosis. (b) Microscopic findings demonstrating acute inflammation and necrosis (hematoxylin and eosin, original magnification ×10). (Source: Adam M. Rotunda. Reproduced with permission of Adam M. Rotunda.)

fibrosis are desirable for localized subcutaneous volume reduction and for promoting tissue tightening. [2, 3, 20].

Under certain conditions, deoxycholate appears to indiscriminately target adipose as well as nonadipose cells and tissue [45, 48, 59, 49, 50]. One study demonstrated that *in vitro*, high-dose (5%) DC, as well as PC (5%)/DC (2.5%), induce necrosis of porcine fat and muscle [45]. Gupta *et al.* [48] showed a cytotoxic response to PC/DC of four different cell types' culture. Jancke [59] also found that Lipostabil had dose-related cytolytic effects on adipose tissue, vascular smooth muscle cells, renal epithelial cells, and myocytes. Schuller-Petrovic [28] found that injection of PC/DC and DC in subcutaneous fat of rats caused fibrosis in adjacent cutaneous muscle.

The proclivity for DC to solubilize adipose, as well as nonadipose cell is unsettling, and would appear to explain skin ulceration in isolated reports [13, 58]. However, in all the reported clinical studies, case series, and FDA registration trials, ulceration with DC is nonexistent. Why the dichotomy? Researchers have recently demonstrated that DC's ability to lyse cells is inversely related to the amount of protein surrounding and within tissue with which it comes into contact, sparing the tissue from necrosis (Figure 4.10) [49]. This effect is mediated in large part by the presence of albumin (an abundant, ubiquitous physiologic protein), which has a very high affinity to DC and appears to inhibit the lytic activity of DC (Figure 4.11) [49]. Therefore, albumin's high concentration in vital tissue but relatively low concentration in fat may explain why injections of deoxycholate into fat are relatively safe clinically. In the available data from Phase 2a and 2b clinical trials [56], which represents safety reporting on over 350 subjects, skin necrosis and damage to other "bystander" tissue by a DC-based medication was not reported. These results are very encouraging.

However, detergent injections are not without temporary downtime. Injection site erythema, tenderness, paresthesias (primarily numbness), and edema are the primary local adverse reactions to DC-injected fat [3, 30, 31, 44, 56]. These effects are generally mild to moderate and dissipate over days to weeks, with no persistent untoward effects. There does appear to be, however, a dose-dependent response to DC, whereby increasing DC concentrations produces increasing degrees of cytotoxicity [45, 48], and subcutaneous fat necrosis [2, 29, 31, 55].

These data collectively suggest some safe therapeutic margin, where maximum benefit is achieved with minimal risk, which is currently being defined and exploited [56]. Factors such as injection technique [2, 35, 46, 60], dose (volume and concentration) [2, 3, 35, 45, 46, 60], and tissue–detergent interactions [3, 19, 60, 50] most likely influence the extent of this "safety window." Some authors suggest that when DC is used without PC, concentrations of the detergent should be less than or equal to 1% [3] as DC greater than 1% is associated with pain, profound tissue necrosis, and prolonged nodularity [2, 30, 31]. Correct injection depth of subcutaneous detergent formulations is also critical [2, 20, 58, 60].

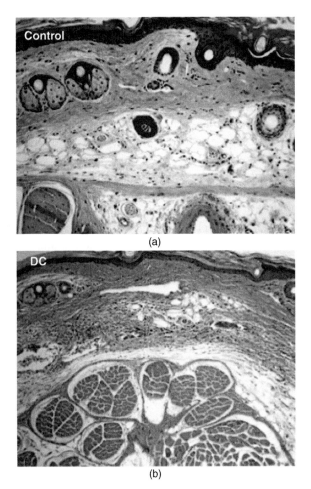

(a)

(b)

Figure 4.10 (a) Hematoxylin and eosin staining of a mouse tail 20 days postinjection of saline vehicle or (b) 0.5% deoxycholate showing necrosis and inflammatory infiltrate of the subcutaneous fat in the treated tail. (b) The tissue architecture of the muscle and skin layers remains preserved in the treated tail, with no signs of necrosis and scant inflammation.

Superficial placement may produce cutaneous breakdown and ulceration [2, 58]. Notably, all reports of scarring and ulceration using detergent-based formulations are associated with nonphysician injectors, large injection volumes, unverified dosages of unknown medications, and other unorthodox practices [8, 13, 58, 60]. As with other injectables, injection technique and practitioner skill and experience are paramount to safety.

An additional question – "what happens to the DC after it is injected?" – has been answered with radioisotope labeled DC injections into fat pads of mice, in an effort to track the body's processing of injected DC [49]. Almost half of the DC injected was transported to the intestinal tract within 24 h of injection

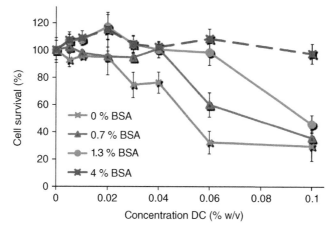

Figure 4.11 Viability of cultured primary human adipocytes treated with deoxycholate (DC) in the presence of increasing concentrations of bovine serum albumin (BSA). Cells were incubated with 0% BSA (orange), 0.7% BSA (blue), 1.3% BSA (green), and 4% BSA (red), and then challenged with increasing concentrations of DC. Cell survival was measured using the 3-(4,5-dimethylthiazol-2-yl)-5-(3-carboxymethoxyphenyl)-2-(4-sulfophenyl)-2H-tetrazolium colorimetric assay for cell viability. The concentrations of bovine serum albumin used are representative of the concentrations found physiologically in and around the site of injection. Albumin attenuated DC-mediated cytolysis in a concentration-dependent manner. Error bars represent standard error of the mean.

into fat tissue. A peak accumulation in the small intestine was noted at 4 h, and at 5 days, the remaining DC was eliminated in the feces. In humans, subcutaneously injected deoxycholate is eliminated from systemic circulation in less than 24 h [56].

The fate of adipolytic therapy

In contrast to the pathway taken by most novel medical therapies (from discovery to preclinical then clinical testing, regulatory approval then product commercialization), it is apparent that before the acquisition of DC by the pharmaceutical industry, the research and clinical experience with injectable detergents was unconventional and haphazard. A pivotal moment in the evolution of this treatment came in 2005, when KYTHERA Biopharmaceuticals (Calabasas, CA) acquired the intellectual rights describing the use of sodium deoxycholate as an injectable fat loss medication from the Los Angeles Biomedical Institute and University of California Los Angeles (UCLA). Since then, the study of detergent-based medication for localized fat loss has been extensive. Preclinical data and clinical registration studies performed by KYTHERA have more clearly characterized the safety and clinical potential of DC, and distinguished it from Lipostabil, PC/DC, and Lipodissolve.

KYTHERA Biopharmaceuticals (Westlake Village, CA), is currently seeking approval of a nonanimal source DC fat-reducing formula for submental fat, referred to as ATX-101; as of this writing, they have entered into Phase 3 (the last phase of clinical drug development before regulatory approval) outside the United States and have just completed Phase 2b testing in the United States. The strategy of using low dose DC (1 or 2 mg/mL) is consistent with prior, nonindustry sponsored investigations, and with the experiences of veteran injectors, who recognize that low dose DC (without PC) is a prudent approach to yield gratifying results while minimizing risks.

A recent Phase 2b, randomized, double-blind, placebo-controlled, dose-ranging study showed ATX-101 was well-tolerated and demonstrated statistically significant efficacy as compared with placebo [56]. The study enrolled a total of 129 subjects and was conducted across 10 dermatology and plastic surgery centers in the United States. Multiple clinician and patient endpoints were assessed as well as magnetic resonance imaging (MRI) to objectively quantify fat reduction. The study tested two drug-dosing regimens (1 and 2 mg/cm^2). In the study, ATX-101 demonstrated statistically significant ($p < 0.05$) reductions in submental fat as compared with placebo as assessed by all measures: a validated clinician scale, patient-reported outcome (PRO) scale, and MRI measurement for both fat volume and thickness. Adverse events (i.e., local swelling, tenderness, erythema) were primarily mild to moderate, and were transient. In addition, a statistically significant difference versus placebo was also shown on other PRO measures, including instruments measuring subject satisfaction, patient impact, and chin attractiveness.

As of this writing, KYTHERA has completed seven clinical trials and treated more than 350 subjects. In two previously conducted ex-US Phase 2 studies on 155 patients, ATX-101 was well-tolerated and yielded statistically significant reduction of submental fat compared to placebo based on clinician and patient assessments. Results observed from their current Phase 2b study confirmed the observations made in previous Phase 2 trials. Phase 3 studies of ATX-101 were initiated in late 2010 in Europe in collaboration with Bayer HealthCare's dermatology unit Intendis, which has licensed rights to ATX-101 outside of the United States and Canada.

LIPO-102 and related lipolytic agents

Using FDA registered drugs, which are proven safe and effective in other indications (i.e., Advair® Discus 5/500, marketed for asthma and COPD, Glaxo-SmithKline), LIPO-102 targets and stimulates adipocyte (intracellular) lipolysis to produce a nonadipolytic, nonsurgical fat tissue reduction. Similar to Advair but in injectable form, LIPO-102 is a combination of salmeterol xinafoate and fluticasone propionate.

Salmeterol xinafoate is a highly selective long-acting β_2-adrenergic receptor agonist. Fluticasone propionate is a synthetic trifluorinated glucocorticoid.

Activation of β_2-adrenergic receptors located on human fat cells by salmeterol triggers the breakdown of triglycerides in these cells to free fatty acids and glycerol by lipolysis. Fluticasone propionate has potent anti-inflammatory activity. Glucocorticoids such as fluticasone impart various effects on β-adrenergic receptor function *in vivo*: they enhance the coupling of β-adrenergic receptors to G proteins and the resulting activation of adenylate cyclase, and they decrease β-adrenergic receptor down-regulation (tachyphylaxis) because of chronic receptor stimulation (e.g., by salmeterol) [61], although tachyphylaxis can be still recognized to some degree clinically. In addition, salmeterol stimulates lipolysis through the activation of β_2-adrenergic receptors on fat cells and fluticasone upregulates the cellular pathways stimulated by salmeterol.

In clinical testing with sophisticated volumetric imaging technology (Canfield Vectra® analysis), 22 weekly abdominal injections of LIPO-102 (0.5 µg salmeterol and 1 µg fluticasone) in 20 subjects for 4–8 weeks produced rapid (within weeks) and significant reductions in abdominal circumference and volume versus placebo (20 subjects). Prior dose escalation studies revealed that higher doses of the combination drugs produced tachyphylaxis and minimal efficacy. Plasma levels of fluticasone and salmeterol produced by LIPO-102 injection are a fraction of those produced by the 505(b)(2) reference drug, Advair 500/50. Anticipated weekly dose is ∼1/700th of Advair weekly dose (based on salmeterol).

At 8 weeks, LIPO-102 produced a mean reduction in abdominal circumference greater than2 cm and a mean reduction in abdominal volume greater than $350\,cm^3$ in young patients. Interestingly, younger subjects (defined as <40 years of age) also had significantly better responses than older subjects; significant reduction in waist circumference relative to placebo only occurred in young subjects (Figure 4.12). Overall change in waist circumference was statistically significant at 6 weeks postdosing, but at the 12-week follow-up, they failed to reach significance. There were no significant hematologic, cardiovascular, or dermatologic adverse effects (i.e., atrophy, pigmentation, nodularity, necrosis). In fact, there was minimal difference in swelling, redness, irritation, or any other local injection site reactions between LIPO-102 and placebo.

Another small but methodologically compelling study provides additional insight into the response of subcutaneous fat to lipolytic compounds [61]. An injected combination of steroid (prednisolone) and a nonselective β-agonist (isoproterenol) produced an average volume decrease of 50% in 10 lipomas injected five times a week for 1 month. There were no acute or chronic adverse effects. All except one of the lipomas, which were measured until 1 year posttreatment, recurred.

It is perhaps too early to tell whether LIPO-102 or any similarly acting lipolytic compound becomes a very useful minimally invasive (injectable) treatment for fat reduction. Ideal injection technique, dosing, and patient selection are still unknown. The data suggests rapid onset after frequent treatment, but some (yet undefined) likelihood of fat reaccumulation several months after treatment.

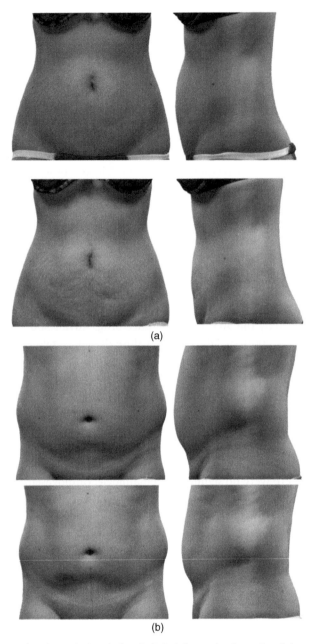

(a)

(b)

Figure 4.12 (a) Before (superior) and after (inferior) 1 month of anterior abdomen injections (one injection session weekly) with 1 μg salmeterol xinafoate and 22 μg fluticasone propionate (total weekly dose) at 8-week follow-up. Volumetric reduction (as measured by Canfield Vectra imaging system): waist reduction: −2.85 cm^3 and volume reduction: −355 cm^3. (b) Before (superior) and after (inferior) 1 month of anterior abdomen injections (one injection session weekly) with 1 μg salmeterol xinafoate and 22 μg fluticasone propionate (total weekly dose) at 8-week follow-up. Volumetric reduction (as measured by Canfield Vectra imaging system): waist reduction: −4.52 cm and volume reduction: −857 cm^3.

Lithera is seeking approval of its drug for anterior abdominal fat reduction, as well as exophthalmos related to retro-orbital fat accumulation. Should the durability of the treatment response be limited only to several months, pharmaceutical lipoplasty may be a boon to aesthetic medicine (recurrent, nonpermanent treatments such as hyaluronic acid tissue fillers and botulinum toxin are the gold standard among injectables). On the other hand, lipolytic agents may fall short if expectations are that any fat treatment, including a simple, "no downtime" injectable, be permanent.

Injectables for cellulite

Cellulite is a psychologically disturbing but physically benign condition. Rotunda and Avram [18] performed an extensive review of the literature about injectables for cellulite several years ago. Our conclusions then remain the same as they are today: until rigorous clinical studies are performed to validate the efficacy of any injectable (including traditional mesotherapy compounds, lipolytic agents, and connective tissue lytic agents), it is unknown whether these agents have any meaningful clinical effect. The only potential treatment entering clinical trials at this point in time is collagenase [62]. As with all the other therapies discussed in this chapter, time and further investigation will determine their ultimate fate.

Conclusions

A safe and effective injectable capable of reducing fat may become available in the near future. Injectable fat-reducing therapies are not an alternative to liposuction or other forms of "body sculpting." Rather, they may be best more appropriately for patients unwilling or unable to have surgical reduction of small collections of fat, or for those patients who desire touch-ups for liposuction-induced irregularities. Extensive preclinical safety testing and rigorous clinical trials demonstrating a favorable product profile using a pharmaceutical grade formulation will be required for regulatory authority approval. Novel lipolytic (LIPO-102) and adipolytic (ATX-101) agents are currently in registration trials. Physicians should avoid compounded, nonregulated medications for the purpose of reducing fat and anticipate the outcome of FDA registered clinical trials shortly.

References

1 Matarasso, A. & Pfeifer, T.M. (2009) Mesotherapy and injection lipolysis. *Clinics in Plastic Surgery*, **36**, 181–192.
2 Duncan, D., Rubin, J.P., Golitz, L. *et al.* (2009) Refinement of technique in injection lipolysis based on scientific studies and clinical evaluation. *Clinics in Plastic Surgery*, **36**, 195–209.

3 Rotunda, A.M., Weiss, S.R. & Rivkin, L.S. (2009) Randomized double-blind clinical trial of subcutaneously injected deoxycholate versus a phosphatidylcholine–deoxycholate combination for the reduction of submental fat. *Dermatologic Surgery*, **35**, 792–803.

4 Atiyeh, B.S., Ibrahim, A.E. & Dibo, S.A. (2008) Cosmetic mesotherapy: between scientific evidence, science fiction, and lucrative business. *Aesthetic Plastic Surgery*, **32**, 842–849.

5 Rotunda, A.M. & Kolodney, M.S. (2006) Mesotherapy and phosphatidylcholine injections: historical clarification and review. *Dermatologic Surgery*, **32**, 465–480.

6 United States Food and Drug Administration (USFDA). (2008) *Statement on lipo dissolve*. Available at: http://www.fda.gov [accessed on 15 June 2009].

7 Carbonne, A., Brossier, F., Arnaud, I. *et al.* (2009) Outbreak of nontuberculous Mycobacteria subcutaneous infections related to multiple mesotherapy injections. *Journal of Clinical Microbiology*, **47**, 1961–1964.

8 Beer, K. & Waibel, J. (2009) Disfiguring scarring following mesotherapy associated *Mycobacterium cosmeticum* infection. *Journal of Drugs in Dermatology*, **8**, 391–393.

9 *Consumer safety alert on fat dissolving injections*. (2007) Available at: http://www.prnewswire.com [accessed on 15 June 2009].

10 American Society for Dermatologic Surgery. (2006) *Emerging technology report: mesotherapy*. Available at: http://www.asds-net.org/Media/ PositionStatements/emerging_technology-mesotherapy.html [accessed on 15 June 2009].

11 American Society for Aesthetic Plastic Surgery. (2007) *American Society for Aesthetic Plastic Surgery warns patients to steer clear of injection fat loss treatments*. Available at: http://www.surgery.org/press/news-release.php?iid1/4475 [accessed on 15 June 2009].

12 Rundle, R.L. Popular treatment that aims to melt fat draws scrutiny. *Wall Street Journal*, 12 June 2007. Available at: http://online.wsj.com/article/SB118160554567831887.html?mod1/4home_health_right [accessed on 15 June 2009].

13 Boodman, S.G. Can shots safely 'melt away fat'? *Washington Post*, Tuesday, 26 June 2007. Available at: http://www.washingtonpost.com/wp-dyn/content/article/2007/06/22/AR2007062201870.html [accessed on 15 June 2009].

14 KCTV 5 News. Lipodissolve company to file bankruptcy, 11 December 2007. Available at: http://www.kctv5.com/news/14822891/detail.html [accessed on 15 June 2009].

15 Rang, H.P., Dale, M.M., Ritter, J.M. *et al.* (2003) *Chapter 11: Pharmacology*. Elsevier Churchill Livingstone, Philadelphia, PA.

16 Motolese, P. (2008) Phospholipids do not have lipolytic activity. A critical review. *Journal of Cosmetic and Laser Therapy*, **10**, 114–118.

17 Greenway, F.L. & Bray, G.A. (1987) Regional fat loss from the thigh in obese women after adrenergic modulation. *Clinical Therapeutics*, **9**, 663–669.

18 Rotunda, A.M., Avram, M.M. & Avram, A.S. (2005) Cellulite: is there a role for injectables? *Journal of Cosmetic and Laser Therapy*, **7**, 147–154.

19 Rotunda, A.M. (2008) Commentary to Schuller-Petrovic *et al.* Tissue-toxic effects of phosphatidylcholine/deoxycholate after subcutaneous injection for fat dissolution in rats and a human volunteer. *Dermatologic Surgery*, **34**, 534–535.

20 Duncan, D. (2005) Lipodissolve for subcutaneous fat reduction and skin retraction. *Aesthetic Surgery Journal* , **25**, 530–543.

21 Pistor, M. (1964) *Mesotherapy*. Librairie Maloine S.A., Paris.

22 Park, S.H., Kim, D.W., Lee, M.A. *et al.* (2008) Effectiveness of mesotherapy on body contouring. *Plastic and Reconstructive Surgery*, **121**, 179e–185e.

23 Lee, J.H., Park, J.G., Lim, S.H. *et al.* (2006) Localized intradermal microinjection of tranexamic acid for treatment of melasma in Asian patients: a preliminary clinical trial. *Dermatologic Surgery*, **32**, 626–631.

24 Cacchio, A., De Blasis, E., Desiati, P. *et al.* (2009) Effectiveness of treatment of calcific tendinitis of the shoulder by disodium EDTA. *Arthritis and Rheumatism*, **15**, 84–91.

25 Lacarrubba, F., Tedeschi, A., Nardone, B. *et al.* (2008) Mesotherapy for skin rejuvenation: assessment of the subepidermal low-echogenic band by ultrasound evaluation with cross-sectional B-mode scanning. *Dermatology and Therapy*, **21**, S1–S5.

26 Amin, S.P., Phelps, R.G. & Goldberg, D.J. (2006) Mesotherapy for facial skin rejuvenation: a clinical, histologic, and electron microscopic evaluation. *Dermatologic Surgery*, **32**, 1467–1472.

27 Rittes, P.G. (2001) The use of phosphatidylcholine for correction of lower lid bulging due to prominent fat pads. *Dermatologic Surgery*, **27**, 391–392.

28 Schuller-Petrovic, S., Wolkart, G., Hofler, G. *et al.* (2008) Tissue-toxic effects of phosphatidylcholine/deoxycholate after subcutaneous injection for fat dissolution in rats and a human volunteer. *Dermatologic Surgery*, **34**, 524–529.

29 Yagina Odo, Y.M.E., Cuce, L.C., Odo, L.M. *et al.* (2007) Action of sodium deoxycholate on subcutaneous human tissue: local and systemic effects. *Dermatologic Surgery*, **33**, 178–188.

30 Salti, G., Ghersetich, I., Tantussi, F. *et al.* (2008) Phosphatidylcholine and sodium deoxycholate in the treatment of localized fat: a double-blind, randomized study. *Dermatologic Surgery*, **34**, 60–66.

31 Rotunda, A.M., Ablon, G. & Kolodney, M.S. (2005) Lipomas treated with subcutaneous deoxycholate injections. *Journal of the American Academy of Dermatology*, **53**, 973–978.

32 Goldman, M.P. (2004) Sodium tetradecyl sulfate for sclerotherapy treatment of veins: is compounding pharmacy solution safe? *Dermatologic Surgery*, **30**, 1454–1456.

33 Rittes, P.G. (2007) Complications of Lipostabil Endova for treating localized fat deposits. *Aesthetic Surgery Journal* , **27**, 146–149.

34 Rittes, P.G., Rittes, J.C. & Carriel Amary, M.F. (2006) Injection of phosphatidylcholine in fat tissue: experimental study of local action in rabbits. *Aesthetic Plastic Surgery*, **30**, 474–478.

35 Rittes, P.G. (2009) The lipodissolve technique: clinical experience. *Clinics in Plastic Surgery*, **36**, 215–221.

36 Hexsel, D.M., Serra, M., de Oliveira, D.'.F.T. *et al.* (2003) Phosphatidylcholine in the treatment of localized fat. *Journal of Drugs in Dermatology*, **2**, 511–518.

37 Treacy, P. & Goldberg, D. (2006) Use of phosphatidylcholine for the correction of lower lid bulging due to prominent fat pads. *Journal of Cosmetic and Laser Therapy*, **8**, 129–132.

38 Hexsel, D.M., Serra, M., de Oliveira Dal'Forno, T. & Zechmeister do Prado, D. (2005) Cosmetic uses of injectable PC on the face. *Otolaryngologic Clinics of North America*, **38**, 1119–1129.

39 Palmer, M., Curran, J. & Bowler, P. (2006) Clinical experience and safety using phosphatidylcholine injections for the localized reduction of subcutaneous fat: a multicentre, retrospective UK study. *Journal of Cosmetic Dermatology*, **5**, 218–226.

40 Bechara, F.G., Sand, M., Hoffmann, K. *et al.* (2007) Fat tissue after lipolysis of lipomas: a histopathological and immunohistochemical study. *Journal of Cutaneous Pathology*, **34**, 552–557.

41 Kopera, D., Binder, B. & Toplak, H. (2006) Intralesional lipolysis with phosphatidylcholine for the treatment of lipomas: pilot study. *Archives of Dermatology*, **142**, 395–396.

42 Myers, P. (2006) The cosmetic use of phosphatidylcholine in the treatment of localized fat deposits. *Cosmetic Dermatology*, **19**, 4120–4160.

43 Ablon, G. & Rotunda, A.M. (2004) Treatment of lower eyelid fat pads using phosphatidylcholine: clinical trial and review. *Dermatologic Surgery*, **30**, 422–427.

44 Rotunda, A.M. & Jones, D.H. (2010) HIV-associated lipohypertrophy (buccal fat-pad lipoma-like lesions) reduced with subcutaneously injected sodium deoxycholate. *Dermatologic Surgery*, **36**, 1348–1354.

45 Rotunda, A.M., Suzuki, H., Moy, R.L. *et al.* (2004) Detergent effects of sodium deoxycholate are a major feature of an injectable phosphatidylcholine formulation used for localized fat dissolution. *Dermatologic Surgery*, **30**, 1001–1008.

46 Duncan, D.I. & Hasengschwandtner, F. (2005) Lipodissolve for subcutaneous fat reduction and skin retraction. *Aesthetic Surgery Journal*, **25**, 530–543.

47 Durr, M., Hager, J. & Lohr, J.P. (1994) Investigations on mixed micelle and liposome preparations for parenteral use based on soya phosphatidylcholine. *European Journal of Pharmaceutics and Biopharmaceutics*, **40**, 147–156.

48 Gupta, A., Lobocki, C., Singh, S. *et al.* (2009) Actions and comparative efficacy of phosphatidylcholine formulation and isolated sodium deoxycholate for different cell types. *Aesthetic Plastic Surgery*, **33**, 346–352.

49 Thuangtong, R., Bentow, J.J., Knopp, K. *et al.* (2010) Tissue-selective effects of injected deoxycholate. *Dermatologic Surgery*, **36**, 899–908.

50 Klein, S.M., Schreml, S., Nerlich, M. *et al.* (2009) In vitro studies investigating the effect of subcutaneous phosphatidylcholine injections in the 3T3-L1 adipocyte model: lipolysis or lipid dissolution? *Plastic and Reconstructive Surgery*, **124**, 419–427.

51 Lichtenberg, D., Zilberman, Y., Greenzaid, P. *et al.* (1979) Structural and kinetic studies on the solubilization of lecithin by sodium deoxycholate. *Biochemistry*, **18**, 3517–3525.

52 Bangham, J.A. & Lea, E.J. (1978) The interaction of detergents with bilayer lipid membranes. *Biochimica et Biophysica Acta*, **511**, 388–396.

53 Lichtenberg, D. (1985) Characterization of the solubilization of lipid bilayers by surfactants. *Biochimica et Biophysica Acta*, **821**, 470–478.

54 Jones, M.N. (1999) Surfactants in membrane solubilisation. *International Journal of Pharmaceutics*, **177**, 137–159.

55 Bentow, J., Suzuki, H., Nahmood, N. *et al.* (2009) Phosphatidylcholine inhibits the adipolytic activity of deoxycholate in vitro and in vivo. *The 5th Continent Congress*. Abstract.

56 Kythera Biopharmaceuticals. Available at: http://www.kytherabiopharma.com/newsroom/ [accessed on 13 February 2011].

57 Tisi, P.V., Beverley, C. & Rees, A. (2006) Injection sclerotherapy for varicose veins. *Cochrane Database of Systematic Reviews*, **4** CD001732.

58 Davis, M.D., Wright, T.I. & Shehan, J.M. (2008) A complication of mesotherapy: noninfectious granulomatous panniculitis. *Archives of Dermatology*, **144**, 808–809.

59 Janke, J., Engeli, S. *et al.* (2009) Compounds used for injection lipolysis destroy adipocytes and other cells found in adipose tissue. *Obesity Facts*, **2**, 36–39.

60 Rotunda, A.M. & Avram, M.M. (2009) The importance of caution in the use of unregulated anticellulite treatments. *Archives of Dermatology*, **145**, 337.

61 Redman, L.M., Moro, C., Dobak, J. *et al.* (2011) Association of beta-2 adrenergic agonist and corticosteroid injection in the treatment of lipomas. *Diabetes, Obesity & Metabolism*, **13**, 517–522.

62 Dagum, A.B. & Badalamente, M.A. (2006) Collagenase injection in the treatment of cellulite. *ASAPS Annual meeting 2006*. Available at: http://asps.confex.com/asps/2006am/techprogram/paper_10359.htm [accessed on 13 February 2011].

CHAPTER 5

The architecture of cellulite

Arisa E. Ortiz[1] and Mathew M. Avram[2]

[1] Division of Dermatology, Laser and Cosmetic Surgery, University of California, CA, USA
[2] Dermatology Laser & Cosmetic Center, Massachusetts General Hospital, MA, USA

Introduction

The term "cellulite" was coined over 150 years ago in the French medical literature [1]. Synonyms for cellulite include adiposis edematosa, status protusus cutis, dermopanniculosis deformans, nodular liposclerosis, gynoid lipodystrophy, and edematofibrosclerotic panniculopathy [2, 3]. Cellulite is a topographic skin change that results in the unattractive cottage cheese-type dimpling of the skin. It can be located in any part of the body containing subcutaneous adipose tissue, but is most commonly seen on the thighs and buttocks [1]. Cellulite can also be found in any pattern of adipose deposition in women, including the breasts, the abdomen, and the arms.

Cellulite is present to some degree in 85–98% of postpubertal women and should be thought of as a women secondary sex characteristic. Cellulite is present in women of all races [4], but it is more prevalent in Caucasian women when compared to Asian women [5]. On the other hand, cellulite is rarely seen in men [1, 6], suggesting a hormonal component to its etiology. A hormonal influence is further supported by the presence of cellulite in men with androgen-deficient states such as Klinefelter's syndrome, hypogonadism, postcastration, and in men receiving estrogen therapy for prostate cancer [7].

It is important to distinguish cellulite from obesity. While obesity is defined as a global increase in adipose tissue from hypertrophy and hyperplasia of adipocytes [8], the characteristic "peau d'orange" appearance of cellulite is generally limited to parts of female pattern adipose distribution. Cellulite can be present in the absence of obesity, as it also occurs in slim individuals [4]. It is rarely seen in men of any weight.

There have been few scientific investigations into the pathophysiology of cellulite. It seems to be multifactorial involving hormonal factors, fat accumulation, microcirculatory dysfunction, altered matrix metabolism, and inflammatory changes [7, 9]. Although cellulite is not a "pathologic" condition associated with any morbidity or mortality [3], it remains an issue of cosmetic concern to a great number of individuals and is of aesthetic significance for that reason. Despite its prevalence, there has been little advancement in our understanding of its pathophysiology. Our limited understanding of the origin and structural composition of cellulite hinders the ability to develop effective treatments. Further investigation of the pathophysiology of cellulite may ultimately lead to more successful treatment modalities.

What defines cellulite?

Several observations between cellulite pathophysiology and "normal" fat have been proposed, but are largely unknown. The four leading hypotheses to explain the physiology of cellulite include sexually dimorphic skin architecture, altered connective tissue septae, vascular changes, and inflammatory factors [7]. However, many other factors seem to play a role in the development of cellulite.

Sexually dimorphic skin architecture

Sexually dimorphic architecture of subcutaneous fat lobules and connective tissue septae has been observed as a leading factor in the development of cellulite. Nürnberger and Müller [4] originally proposed that the appearance of cellulite dimpling was a result of herniations of fat, termed "papillae adiposae," that protrude through a weakened dermis. Fat herniations into the dermis have been visualized by ultrasound imaging as low-density, hyperechoic regions between denser, hypoechoic dermal tissues [10]. Sonographic imaging of women has shown an uneven and discontinuous dermo-hypodermal interface representing fat herniations into the dermis. In contrast, male anatomy exhibits a smooth and continuous dermo-hypodermal junction. However, this gender-related difference is not localized to affected areas of cellulite. Rather, fat herniation is considered to be a diffuse finding seen in women regardless of the clinical evidence of cellulite. Another finding seen in affected women on ultrasound is thinner dermal septae arranged perpendicular to the dermal surface. This is thought to facilitate the protrusion of the fat lobules into the reticular dermis. In comparison, thicker septae that are arranged obliquely to the dermis are seen in men, who rarely display cellulite. The thickness of the septae in men and women seen with ultrasound imaging has been confirmed by more advanced techniques such as magnetic resonance imaging (MRI).

MRI has improved the imaging capabilities for evaluating differences in architecture between areas of cellulite compared to "normal" fat. MRI actually demonstrates thicker fibrous septae in cellulite areas when compared to "normal" areas [11]. Other MRI findings have shown a great increase in the thickness of the inner (lamellar) fat layer in women with cellulite in addition to a higher percentage of tortuous septae oriented in a direction perpendicular to the skin surface [12]. Men and women without cellulite were more likely to have septae parallel to the skin or angulated to 45° presumably creating a more supportive structure resistant to herniation. Interestingly, spectroscopy in these patients did not detect any differences in the unsaturated lipid fraction, the saturated lipid fraction, or the water fraction between the fat lobules in men compared to women, or in cellulite versus "normal" fat. Thus, discrediting the theory that excess water content in the adipose tissue of women plays a role in the development of cellulite.

Altered connective tissue septae

The Nürnberger and Müller hypothesis [4] has been debated by subsequent studies, which have not correlated the presence of cellulite with fatty protrusions through the dermal–hypodermal interface. Similar to ultrasound findings, studies of autopsy specimens have shown a smooth dermo-hypodermal interface on microscopic examination of unaffected men [13]. Women were associated with the presence of papillae adiposae herniating into the undersurface of the dermis. There was no association, however, between the extent of these protrusions and the clinical severity of cellulite. A distinguishing feature between cellulite-prone skin and unaffected skin was found to be uneven thickness of connective tissue septae, showing a few α-actin-positive myofibroblasts in thicker points. These findings are consistent with previous studies that show a distinct difference in the structure of the hypodermis in the thighs and in the buttocks between men and women. Again, this difference seems to be irrelevant to the extent of the appearance of cellulite clinically. Instead, full-blown cellulite (overt dimpling of the skin without manipulation) is thought to be a result of stretching from vertical fibrous strands that are oriented perpendicular to the skin, allowing fat herniation through the weakened connective tissue buttress.

Vascular changes

It has been suggested that the development of cellulite begins with the deterioration of the dermal vasculature [14, 15]. Specifically, dysfunction of the dermal precapillary arteriolar sphincter and deposition of glycosaminoglycans (GAGs) in the capillary walls and within the ground substance leads to a buildup of capillary pressure. Increased capillary pressure results in increased capillovenular permeability leading to extravasation of fluid and retention of fluid exacerbated by further attraction of water within the dermis by hydrophilic GAGs. Chronic edema results in tissue hypoxia from vascular compression, vessel dilatation, and decreased venous return. Tissue hypoxia and deposition of GAGs in dermal collagen and elastic fibers stimulates fibroplasia, collagenesis, and capillary neogenesis. Eventually, chronic edema, vascular congestion, and hypoxia lead to thickened and sclerotic fibrous septae causing the appearance of cellulite. The contribution of vascular compromise to the pathogenesis of cellulite has been debated [1, 4, 13].

Inflammatory factors

Another theory purports that inflammation generates the appearance of cellulite. Macrophages and lymphocytes have been reported in the fibrous septae on biopsy specimens of apparent cellulite [16]. The septae are thought to be the source of chronic inflammation leading to dermal atrophy and adipolysis. A subjective finding that supports the role of inflammation is the feeling of tenderness reported with compression of cellulite [1]. The role of inflammation has not been proven yet and many patients have cellulite without evidence for inflammation or adipolysis [1, 4, 13].

Gender differences in lipid metabolism

Subcutaneous fat is composed of two layers separated by a superficial fascia: an external layer (areolar layer) and a deeper layer (lamellar layer). The areolar layer consists of vertically oriented globular large adipocytes, while the lamellar layer has horizontally arranged smaller adipocytes with larger and more blood vessels [17]. The areolar layer is thicker in women and in children, especially in the femoral region [2].

Adipose tissue is regulated by catecholamines (epinephrine and norepinephrine), which are lipolytic, and insulin, which is antilipolytic. Catecholamine regulation of fat metabolism involves andrenergic receptor (AR) stimulation of adenylate cyclase via lipolytic receptors (β-ARs) and inhibition by antilipolytic receptors (α-2 ARs) [18]. Adipose tissue in different regions of the body behaves differently in response to hormones and metabolic activity. For example, visceral fat is more responsive to catecholamine-stimulated lipolysis than abdominal fat [19, 20]. On the other hand, adipocytes in the gluteofemoral region are larger, more abundant, and appear to be more resistant to lipolysis [20]. This is secondary to the influence of estrogen, which increases the response of adipocytes to antilipolytic α-2 ARs [19]. In general, both sexes are more resistant to lipolysis in gluteofemoral adipocytes compared to abdominal adipocytes. However, men tend to have an android distribution (upper body) of fat and women tend to have a gynoid distribution (lower body) [21–23].

Hormonal differences between men and women likely play a role in the different adipocyte responses to fat metabolism. Men tend to accumulate more fat in the abdominal region, which is suggested to be secondary to increased abdominal antilipolytic α-2 ARs compared to women [18, 20, 24]. Women have greater fatty tissue development in puberty compared to men, likely influenced by estrogen, specifically 17-β-estradiol, which stimulates adipocyte replication [25]. The gluteal region has a higher density of α-2 ARs compared to the abdominal adipocytes, which partially explains the difference in responsiveness to catecholamines in these regions. Additionally, abdominal adipocytes are more responsive to isoproteronol, a β-AR agonist [21, 22]. This mechanism explains the increased sensitivity to catecholamine-induced lipolysis in abdominal fat versus gluteal adipocytes.

Abdominal adipocytes in postmenopausal women are larger and have more abundant β-AR suggested by catecholamine-induced lipolysis, measured by localized lipoprotein lipase (LPL) release [22, 23]. Interestingly, more abundant α-2 ARs are found in gluteal adipocytes of premenopausal and postmenopausal women who are undergoing estrogen replacement therapy. Estrogen plays many roles in fat metabolism and the appearance of cellulite including proliferation of fibroblasts, increase in hyaluronic acid, and increased vascular permeability, leading to edema and fibrosclerosis of connective tissue septae, and increased lipogenesis via stimulation of LPL. Prolactin and thyroid hormones also have a role in adipose tissue development [2].

What type of fat is cellulite made of?

Humans contain both white adipose tissue (WAT) and brown adipose tissue (BAT) to some degree. WAT appears yellow or ivory in color and functions to store excess energy in the form of lipid, which is mobilized in times of metabolic need [26]. BAT appears brown and its function is to use lipids to convert to chemical energy to heat [27, 28]. The brown appearance of BAT is due to a dense vascular network that is associated with mitochondria [29]. BAT and WAT work in opposition to regulate energy metabolism and both are innervated by the noradrenergic sympathetic nervous system. It has been well established that WAT functions in lipid metabolism, glucose metabolism, and endocrine functions [30]. More recent research is challenging the belief that BAT is merely vestigial remnants from the neonatal period [27, 31–33].

Mature adipocytes make up one-third of adipose tissue and the remaining two-thirds are composed of small blood vessels, nerves, fibroblasts, and adipocyte precursors. Mature adipocytes are either of the white or brown cytotype. Among differences in color, white and brown adipocytes are histologically distinct [34].

White adipocytes are organized within one "unilocular" droplet, which can exceed 50 µm in size. They are spherical in shape, allowing for maximal volume expansion in the least amount of space. The nuclei are pushed to one side because of the high lipid content. In comparison, brown adipocytes are smaller (20–40 µm) and are arranged into "mutilocular" droplets. They are polygonal with centrally located nuclei.

WAT and BAT are generally distributed in distinct anatomic locations. WAT can be found in the visceral adipose tissue (intraperitoneal and retroperitoneal) and subcutaneous adipose tissue (superficial and deep). In neonates, BAT is found around blood vessels, in the interscapular region, nape of the neck, axillae, trachea, esophagus, and organs such as the pancreas, adrenal glands, and kidneys [30, 35–37]. In adult humans, there are very few collections of BAT because of a morphologic change from rapid fat accumulation in which they appear more "unilocular" [32].

These distribution patterns are based solely on histologic findings. However, morphology of adipocytes is not always sufficient to differentiate WAT from BAT. For example, brown adipocytes may appear "unilocular" when not being stimulated [32]. Similarly, as white adipocytes lose lipids in fasting states, their morphology can change into a more elongated and "multilocular appearance" [29]. More advanced techniques to detect the presence of uncoupling protein-1 (UCP-1), unique to brown adipocytes, are a more accurate method for identifying activated brown adipocytes [30]. Through polymerase chain reaction or Northern blot hybridization, UCP-1 mRNA has detected scattered brown adipocytes within traditional WAT depots [38, 39]. Furthermore, the previous belief that stem cells are committed to either a white or brown cell lineage has been refuted by transdifferentiation of white adipocytes into brown adipocytes under certain conditions [40, 41]. However, the physiological significance of these findings has yet to be elucidated. These novel techniques are potential avenues to further investigate the composition of cellulite and improve our understanding of how to approach treatment.

Other factors

While obesity does not cause cellulite, weight gain does make cellulite more clinically apparent by increasing the volume of adipocytes. Studies have also found a positive correlation with cellulite and higher body mass index (BMI) [42]. Individuals with a higher BMI have increased extrusion of adipose tissue through the hypodermis because of a thinner dermis and a weakened connective tissue structure. Cellulite is also aggravated by stress, a sedentary lifestyle, and hormonal birth control pills [2]. A sedentary lifestyle may lead to alterations in the microcirculation of cellulite-prone areas through stasis and further impediment of blood flow, not to mention decreased caloric output. Excessive consumption of carbohydrates leads to hyperinsulinemia, which increases total body fat content via lipogenesis. Pregnancy may also promote cellulite by lipogenesis and fluid retention in association with an increase in prolactin, insulin, fluid volume, and lower extremity venous congestion [17]. Even a genetic susceptibility to cellulite has been suggested in a recent study implicating angiotensin I converting enzyme (ACE) and hypoxia-inducible factor-1 alpha (HIF1A) [43].

Conclusion

In summary, the pathophysiology of cellulite remains an enigma. Owing to a lack of understanding of the multifaceted physiology of cellulite, currently available treatments are unsuccessful [44]. Available treatment options are based on anecdotal evidence that generally addresses only one aspect of cellulite. With increasing technology and further investigation, the pathogenesis of cellulite will be further elucidated. Better understanding will lead to improved treatments that address not only structural aspects, but also biochemical factors, as well.

References

1 Scherwitz, C. & Braun-Falco, O. (1978) So-called cellulite. *Journal of Dermatologic Surgery and Oncology*, **4** (**3**), 230–234.
2 Rossi, A.B. & Vergnanini, A.L. (2000) Cellulite: a review. *Journal of the European Academy of Dermatology and Venereology*, **14** (**4**), 251–262.
3 Lotti, T., Ghersetich, I., Grappone, C. & Dini, G. (1990) Proteoglycans in so-called cellulite. *International Journal of Dermatology*, **29** (**4**), 272–274.
4 Nürnberger, F. & Müller, G. (1978) So-called cellulite: an invented disease. *Journal of Dermatologic Surgery and Oncology*, **4** (**3**), 221–229.
5 Draelos, Z.D. (2001) In search of answers regarding cellulite. *Cosmetic Dermatology*, **14**, 55–58.
6 Draelos, Z.D. & Marenus, K.D. (1997) Cellulite. Etiology and purported treatment. *Dermatologic Surgery*, **23** (**12**), 1177–1181.
7 Avram, M.M. (2004) Cellulite: a review of its physiology and treatment. *Journal of Cosmetic and Laser Therapy*, **6** (**4**), 181–185.
8 Bray, G.A. (1989) Obesity: basic considerations and clinical approaches. *Disease-a-Month*, **35** (**7**), 449–537.
9 Rawlings, A.V. (2006) Cellulite and its treatment. *International Journal of Cosmetic Science*, **28** (**3**), 175–190.
10 Rosenbaum, M., Prieto, V., Hellmer, J. *et al.* (1998) An exploratory investigation of the morphology and biochemistry of cellulite. *Plastic and Reconstructive Surgery*, **101** (**7**), 1934–1939.
11 Hexsel, D.M., Abreu, M., Rodrigues, T.C., Soirefmann, M., do Prado, D.Z. & Gamboa, M.M. (2009) Side-by-side comparison of areas with and without cellulite depressions using magnetic resonance imaging. *Dermatologic Surgery*, **35** (**10**), 1471–1477.
12 Querleux, B., Cornillon, C., Jolivet, O. & Bittoun, J. (2002) Anatomy and physiology of subcutaneous adipose tissue by in vivo magnetic resonance imaging and spectroscopy: relationships with sex and presence of cellulite. *Skin Research and Technology*, **8** (**2**), 118–124.

13 Pierard, G.E., Nizet, J.L. & Pierard-Franchimont, C. (2000) Cellulite: from standing fat herniation to hypodermal stretch marks. *American Journal of Dermatopathology*, **22** (**1**), 34–37.
14 Curri, S.B. (1993) Cellulite and fatty tissue microcirculation. *Cosmetics & Toiletries*, **108**, 151–158.
15 Curri, S.B. & Bombardelli, E. (1994) Local lipodystrophy and districtual micro-circulation. *Cosmetics & Toiletries*, **109**, 51–65.
16 Kligman, A. (1997) Cellulite: facts and fiction. *Journal of Geriatric dermatology*, **5**, 136–139.
17 Khan, M.H., Victor, F., Rao, B. & Sadick, N.S. (2010) Treatment of cellulite: part I. Pathophysiology. *Journal of the American Academy of Dermatology*, **62** (**3**), 361–370; quiz 371–362.
18 Leibel, R.L., Edens, N.K. & Fried, S.K. (1989) Physiologic basis for the control of body fat distribution in humans. *Annual Review of Nutrition*, **9**, 417–443.
19 Berlan, M., Galitzky, J. & Lafontan, M. (1992) Hétérogénéité fonctionnelle du tissue adipeux: recepteurs adrenergiques et lipomobilisation. *Le Journal de Médecine Esthétique et de Chirurgie Dermatologique*, **19**, 7–15.
20 Leibel, R.L. & Hirsch, J. (1987) Site- and sex-related differences in adrenoreceptor status of human adipose tissue. *Journal of Clinical Endocrinology and Metabolism*, **64** (**6**), 1205–1210.
21 Mauriege, P., Galitzky, J., Berlan, M. & Lafontan, M. (1987) Heterogeneous distribution of beta and alpha-2 adrenoceptor binding sites in human fat cells from various fat deposits: functional consequences. *European Journal of Clinical Investigation*, **17** (**2**), 156–165.
22 Berman, D.M., Nicklas, B.J., Rogus, E.M., Dennis, K.E. & Goldberg, A.P. (1998) Regional differences in adrenoceptor binding and fat cell lipolysis in obese, postmenopausal women. *Metabolism*, **47** (**4**), 467–473.
23 Ley, C.J., Lees, B. & Stevenson, J.C. (1992) Sex- and menopause-associated changes in body-fat distribution. *American Journal of Clinical Nutrition*, **55** (**5**), 950–954.
24 Wahrenberg, H., Lonnqvist, F. & Arner, P. (1989) Mechanisms underlying regional differences in lipolysis in human adipose tissue. *Journal of Clinical Investigation*, **84** (**2**), 458–467.
25 Krotkiewski, M., Bjorntorp, P., Sjostrom, L. & Smith, U. (1983) Impact of obesity on metabolism in men and women. Importance of regional adipose tissue distribution. *Journal of Clinical Investigation*, **72** (**3**), 1150–1162.
26 Ramsay, T.G. (1996) Fat cells. *Endocrinology and Metabolism Clinics of North America*, **25** (**4**), 847–870.
27 Cannon, B. & Nedergaard, J. (2004) Brown adipose tissue: function and physiological significance. *Physiological Reviews*, **84** (**1**), 277–359.
28 Lowell, B.B. (1998) Adaptive thermogenesis: turning on the heat. *Current Biology*, **8** (**15**), R517–R520.
29 Cinti, S. (2005) The adipose organ. *Prostaglandins, Leukotrienes, and Essential Fatty Acids*, **73** (**1**), 9–15.
30 Avram, A.S., Avram, M.M. & James, W.D. (2005) Subcutaneous fat in normal and diseased states: 2. Anatomy and physiology of white and brown adipose tissue. *Journal of the American Academy of Dermatology*, **53** (**4**), 671–683.
31 Cunningham, S., Leslie, P., Hopwood, D. *et al.* (1985) The characterization and energetic potential of brown adipose tissue in man. *Clinical Science (London)*, **69** (**3**), 343–348.
32 Himms-Hagen, J. (2001) Does brown adipose tissue (BAT) have a role in the physiology or treatment of human obesity? *Reviews in Endocrine & Metabolic Disorders*, **2** (**4**), 395–401.
33 Sell, H., Deshaies, Y. & Richard, D. (2004) The brown adipocyte: update on its metabolic role. *International Journal of Biochemistry and Cell Biology*, **36** (**11**), 2098–2104.
34 Fawcett, D.W. (1952) A comparison of the histological organization and cytochemical reactions of brown and white adipose tissues. *Journal of Morphology*, **90** (**2**), 363–405.
35 Lean, M.E. (1989) Brown adipose tissue in humans. *Proceedings of the Nutrition Society*, **48** (**2**), 243–256.

36 Okuyama, C., Ushijima, Y., Kubota, T. *et al.* (2003) 123I-Metaiodobenzylguanidine uptake in the nape of the neck of children: likely visualization of brown adipose tissue. *Journal of Nuclear Medicine*, **44** (**9**), 1421–1425.

37 Fukuchi, K., Ono, Y., Nakahata, Y., Okada, Y., Hayashida, K. & Ishida, Y. (2003) Visualization of interscapular brown adipose tissue using (99m)Tc-tetrofosmin in pediatric patients. *Journal of Nuclear Medicine*, **44** (**10**), 1582–1585.

38 Garruti, G. & Ricquier, D. (1992) Analysis of uncoupling protein and its mRNA in adipose tissue deposits of adult humans. *International Journal of Obesity and Related Metabolic Disorders*, **16** (**5**), 383–390.

39 Oberkofler, H., Dallinger, G., Liu, Y.M., Hell, E., Krempler, F. & Patsch, W. (1997) Uncoupling protein gene: quantification of expression levels in adipose tissues of obese and non-obese humans. *Journal of Lipid Research*, **38** (**10**), 2125–2133.

40 Tiraby, C., Tavernier, G., Lefort, C. *et al.* (2003) Acquirement of brown fat cell features by human white adipocytes. *J Biol Chem*, **278** (**35**), 33370–33376.

41 Hansen, J.B., te Riele, H. & Kristiansen, K. (2004) Novel function of the retinoblastoma protein in fat: regulation of white versus brown adipocyte differentiation. *Cell Cycle*, **3** (**6**), 774–778.

42 Mirrashed, F., Sharp, J.C., Krause, V., Morgan, J. & Tomanek, B. (2004) Pilot study of dermal and subcutaneous fat structures by MRI in individuals who differ in gender, BMI, and cellulite grading. *Skin Research and Technology*, **10** (**3**), 161–168.

43 Emanuele, E., Bertona, M. & Geroldi, D. (2010) A multilocus candidate approach identifies ACE and HIF1A as susceptibility genes for cellulite. *Journal of the European Academy of Dermatology and Venereology*, **24** (**8**), 930–935.

44 Wanner, M. & Avram, M. (2008) An evidence-based assessment of treatments for cellulite. *Journal of Drugs in Dermatology*, **7** (**4**), 341–345.

CHAPTER 6

Cellulite treatment

Neil S. Sadick[1] and Suveena Bhutani[2]

[1] Weill Cornell Medical College, Cornell University, NY, USA
[2] Sadick Dermatology and Research, NY, USA

There is an increasing demand for the treatment of cellulite, which is considered a common cosmetic condition experienced by more than 90% of women after puberty. For women, the media and western culture continually impress the perfect body image and shape that is free of cellulite. Cellulite is a common topographical alteration, which is defined as a localized metabolic disorder of subcutaneous tissue that provokes an alteration in normal skin morphology. Cellulite is also known by other names, including gynoid lypodystroophy and edematofibrosclerotic panniculopathy. It is physically expressed by skin dimpling and nodularity that occurs mainly in women in the pelvic region, lower limbs, and abdomen and can be seen basically anywhere else where subcutaneous

Fat removal: Invasive and non-invasive body contouring, First Edition. Edited by Mathew M. Avram.
© 2015 John Wiley & Sons, Ltd. Published 2015 by John Wiley & Sons, Ltd.

tissue is found. It is considered as being a secondary sex characteristic, as it is experienced in women after puberty, which is a degenerative occurrence that provokes alterations to the hypodermis, producing irregular undulations on the skin overlying the affected areas manifested as an orange peel or dimpling of the skin (Figures 6.1 and 6.2).

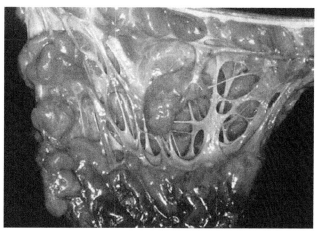

Figure 6.1 Autopsy of amputated leg. Complex network of hypodermal fibrous strands in cellulite. Their thickness is uneven. There is no real septum partitioning the fat lobules. (Source: Pierard *et al.*, 2000 [1]. Reproduced with permission of Lippincott Williams & Wilkins.)

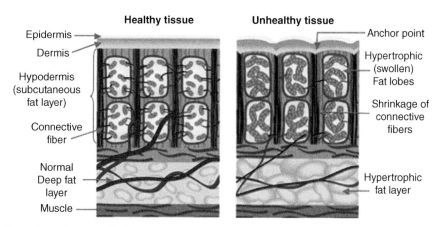

Figure 6.2 Schematic of cellulite.

A clear distinction must be made between cellulite and obesity. Both conditions can occur simultaneously, as obesity encompasses an increase in the subcutaneous fat tissue and can then aggravate the appearance of cellulite. Yet, the etiology of the two conditions is very unique. Hypertrophy and hyperplasia of adipose fat tissue throughout the body characterize obesity, whereas in cellulite it is usually located in the glutei and bitrochanteric regions and usually the resultant of several ultrastructural, inflammatory, histochemical, and morphological changes that produce the distorted and uneven skin.

Scientific discussions in cellulite are fairly new, with the causes of origins of this condition still yet to be scientifically proven. However, several observations and theories have led to proposed etiologies. Genetic predisposition, hormones, inflammation, microcirculatory changes, adipose tissue difference, sexually dimorphic skin architecture, and lifestyle considerations are all thought to result in the formation of cellulite (Figure 6.3) [2]. Treatment approaches for most postpubertal cellulite in women therefore have been highly varied with subjective results (Table 6.1). This chapter discusses the treatment of cellulite by considering patient selection and expected benefits of cellulite treatment, including the latest innovations in noninvasive cellulite technology.

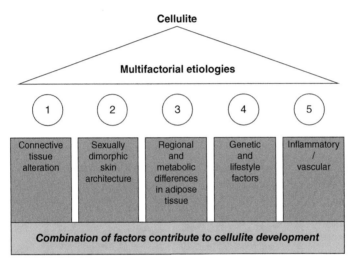

Figure 6.3 Multifactorial etiologies.

Brief overview of cellulite

Cellulite is considered a condition of multifactorial etiology, despite genetics and inherent characteristics playing a vital role in the development of cellulite. These multifactorial etiologies include the following. (1) Sex/gender – the typical pattern of cellulite affects only women. (2) Race – Caucasian women are found to have more cellulite development than women of Asian or African descent. (3) Diet/nutrition – a diet rich in high carbohydrates foods can illicit hyperinsulinmeia and lipogensis yielding an overall increase in total body fat

Table 6.1 Modalities employed in the treatment of cellulite.

Weight loss
Endermologie – suction massage
Liposuction
Subscision – shearing fat septa
Mesotherapy (phosphatidylcholine, caffeine, aminophylline, theophylline, etc.)
Bipolar and unipolar RF devices
Ultrasound
Laser and light sources
Retinoic acid topical application
Carboxytherapy

Table 6.2 Grading of cellulite.

Definition	Grade
Smooth surface of skin while lying down and standing	0
Wrinkles on pinch test	
Smooth surface of skin while lying down and standing	1
Mattress phenomenon on pinch test	
Smooth surface of skin while lying down	
Mattress phenomenon spontaneously while standing	2
Mattress phenomenon spontaneously while standing and lying down	3

content, thereby enhancing cellulite production. (4) Lifestyle – a sedentary lifestyle in which there are prolonged periods of sitting or standing can stunt normal blood flow and can result in stasis and alterations in the microcirculation in the cellulite-prone regions of the body. (5) Pregnancy – it is associated with an increase in particular hormones such as prolactin and insulin and increased fluid volume throughout the body (Table 6.2). Together these factors create lipogenesis and fluid retention stimulating cellulite production.

Cellulite anatomy

The alterations that characterize cellulite are significant depressions that have the same color and consistency as the surrounding normal skin. There is variability in the number of lesions as well as the shapes, such as rounded, oval, or linear. Commonly, cellulite is found in the oval shape and located in the lower buttocks and upper thighs. These sites are more typically aggravated with the aging process, as more flaccidity of the epidermis accumulates. Remarkably, cellulite can be seen to reduce or even disappear on surgically lifting the buttocks to their original position.

When considering cellulite anatomically, it is characterized by topical alterations in the skin, which appear as nodularity and skin dimpling usually as a result of the herniation of subcutaneous fat located in the fibrous connective tissue. The connective tissue of the reticular dermis is connected to the deep fasica by means of fibrous septa from adipose tissue. The fibrous septa are thin rigid strands of connective tissue that intersect the adipose layer and connect the dermis to the underlying fasica, therefore separating the subcutaneous fat lobules from one another [1]. The fibrous septa are vital to stabilizing and dividing the fat. Fibrosis can cause a shortening of the septa, which can provoke an inward pull or retraction at the insertion points of the trabeculas, causing the characteristic depression in cellulite.

In the study of anatomy and histology of fat and connective tissue structure of the subcutaneous tissue by Nurberger and Muller [3], cellulite was described by the term panniculosis of the dermis. Anatomical tests demonstrated the character aspect of cellulite and suggested the differences in the structure pattern in both genders. A perpendicular orientation of the fibrous septa was shown in women in relation to the cutaneous surface, whereas in men there was a crisscross pattern (Figure 6.4).

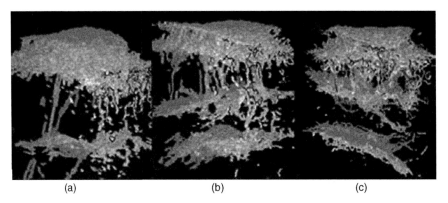

(a)   (b)   (c)

Figure 6.4 Visualization of the 3D architecture of fibrous septae in subcutaneous adipose tissue. (a) a woman with cellulite (b) a woman without cellulite (c) a man. (Source: Querleux *et al.*, 2002 [4]. Reproduced with permission of Wiley.)

Cellulite grading

Various classifications have been developed to classify cellulite, including a common system that classifies cellulite into four different stages or degrees. This was created by Curri [5] on the basis of the pinch test or muscle contraction at rest. Absence of cellulite was labeled Stage 0, while Stage I was defined by smooth skin without any dumpling on standing or lying down but exhibits a mattress-like pattern on skin pinching. This occurs because fat is forced into the dermis on pinching. Stage II is described by visible cellulite on standing but disappearing when the patient is in the supine position. In Stage III, cellulite can be seen in individuals who exhibit skin dimpling on standing, as well as in the supine position, and can be provoked (Table 6.2).

Approach to a patient with cellulite

It is crucial for the physician to discuss the concerns of the patient and their desire to undergo cosmetic rejuvenation. All options for treatment, including the number of visits required, benefits, and side effects should be discussed. Particularly, the importance of false expectations on the part of the patient needs to be addressed; in this case, the physician must stress realistic clinical outcomes and the possibility that a treatment course has little or no results. Those patients whose expectations exceed the realistic results of the procedure must abstain from any course of treatment.

It is imperative analogous to any other health concern or pathology that a thorough medical history be taken by the physician. Questions to be asked include the age of onset of cellulite; previous history of trauma, liposuction, or injections to the affected area; prior illness/surgery; family history including chronic vascular problems or associate hormonal diseases; and all previous and current medications, particularly including any hormone therapy.

A complete physical examination should be conducted, with the patient in a relaxed standing position (Figure 6.5) [6]. It is noted that cellulite can be successfully noted by the pinch test (Figure 6.6), by which skin is pinched between the thumb and index finger to form a fold, or asking the patient to contract the muscle in the observed area [7]. It is suggested to conduct the examination under appropriate overhead lighting to accurately see the cellulite. Elasticity of the skin and subcutaneous tissues can be performed by palpation, although no distinct parameters have been set for classification of skin elasticity. Any health problems related to venous or lymphatic drainage insufficiency may exacerbate cellulite, and this should be evaluated for during the history and physical examination [8]. An examination with a duplex ultrasound of the superficial venous system will be able to confirm and classify the significance of venous insufficiency and direct treatment. On completion of the examination, a localized examination of cellulite areas is performed by inspecting and classifying cellulite areas, checking for edema, lipoedema, or lipolymphoedema. It is important for the physician to also evaluate for lipodystrophy and localized adiposity.

During the initial visit, as well as after each treatment course, it is imperative for photographs to be taken. To better assess and monitor the progress of clinical outcomes, it is always recommended to photograph each visit in the same manner, particularly a whole body image and a close-up photograph of areas

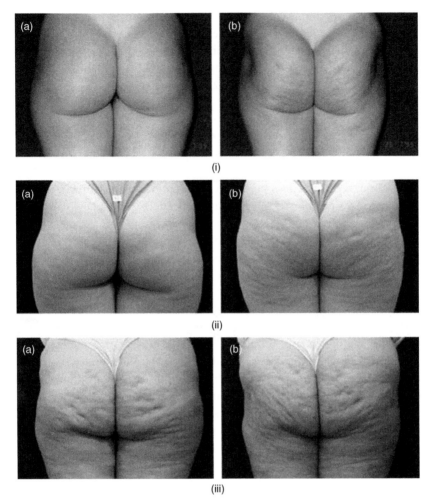

Figure 6.5 Cellulite grade at grade II (i), grade III (ii), and grade 4 (iii) at rest (a) and after gluteal contraction (b). (Source: Rossi *et al.*, (2000) [6]. Reproduced with permission of Wiley.)

being targeted for treatment. Before treatment and after patient consent forms are signed, baseline body weight, BMI calculations, and measurements of circumferential thigh, hip, and/or girth should be taken.

Recent advances and controversies in cellulite treatment

There has been a significant evolution in the area of cellulite technology, and many treatment options are available. These treatment modalities can be found

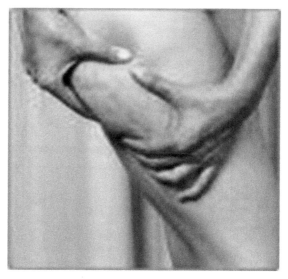

Figure 6.6 The pinch test for cellulite evaluation.

to be separated in three categories, including attenuation of aggravating factors such as weight loss, topically applied pharmacological agents, and interventional methods such as physical, mechanical, and thermal modes of lipolysis and connective tissue alterations. This chapter focuses on the thermal mode of cellulite treatment, more specifically technologies that use laser and light sources for cellulite attenuation.

The effectiveness and validity of a treatment option can be based on many factors, including frequency, length of procedure, total number of treatments required, power levels, and the intensity of vacuum, the mechanical effort, and skill of the operator. When applying device using optical energy and/or optical energy and radiofrequency (RF) and other energy sources, it is noted that their therapeutic effect begins to decrease at about 3 months after treatment. At 6 months, most benefits are reversed, and it is advisable to follow-up with maintenance treatment no later than 6 months [9].

As there is a continual demand for the latest and most effective treatment to eradicate cellulite and fat, many options will be available that use unique method of technology and energy sources. A further discussion of the current devices available is given in this chapter.

TriActive in the treatment of cellulite

Triactive (Cynosure, Westford, MA; Figure 6.7) has three major components to treat cellulite. These three mechanisms include contact cooling, massage,

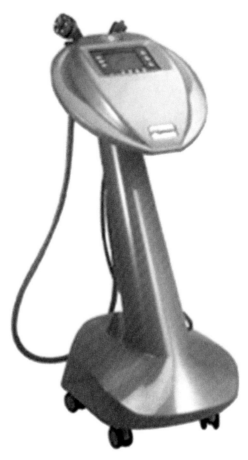

Figure 6.7 TriActive platform. (Source: Cynosure, Westford, MA. Reproduced with permission of Cynosure.)

and diode lasers. The contact cooling system decreases edema by causing vasoconstriction followed by compensatory vasodilatation, allowing the pooled fluid to remobilize. The rhythmic massage counteracts circulatory stasis again by stimulating lymphatic drainage. Six 808-nm diode lasers (Figure 6.8) work directly on the endothelial cells in the vasculature, stimulating arterial, venous, and lymphatic flow, as well as neovascularization [10].

TriActive creates the effects of negative pressure massage present, resulting in stimulation of metabolism, vascularization, and purification via lymphatic drainage [11]. The stretching and rhythmic compression of connective tissue activate fat lobules to cause their shrinkage with stretching of the fibrous septae [12]. It is postulated that the mechanical stimulation is thought to act on the mechanoreceptors in the skin. The excessive distension of subcutaneous tissue activates the specific receptors to free substances such as bradykinin,

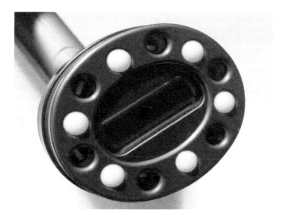

Figure 6.8 TriActive handpiece. (Source: Cynosure, Westford, MA. Reproduced with permission of Cynosure.)

histamine, serotonin, and catecholamines. Lipolysis is mediated by the effect of catecholamines on the beta-adrenergic receptors (β-AR). Activation of β-AR results in the activation of adenocyclase, resulting in an increase in adenosine monophosphate (AMP) and thus an increase in overall tissue AMP concentration. AMP acts as a second messenger and in turn stimulates adipose tissue kinase called adipose tissue lipoprotein lipase (LPL). This intra-adipocytic lipase acts via hydrolytic action on triglycerides of fat cells [13].

TriActive was initially studied in Europe by Nicola Zerbinati [14], in which, 10 patients were treated with 20-min sessions three times a week. Clinical observations, circumference of the thighs and hips, plicometry, skin elasticity, and thermography were recorded. All patients showed an improvement in skin tone and a reduction in the circumference of the areas treated.

The motivation for the use of diode laser is based on the work by Schindl *et al.* who documented increased dermal angiogenesis after treatment with a diode laser therapy [10]. In addition, previous groups have reported increased levels of procollagen I and III mRNA after treatment with low intensity laser irradiation [15]. In a study evaluated by Frew and Katz [16], 10 female patients, aged 18–60 years with moderate cellulite bilaterally were treated with TriActive. All patients were treated biweekly for a total of 16 treatments. Half of the affected body area was treated with the diode laser, contact cooling, and suction operation, per standard TriActive treatment, whereas the contralateral side was treated with the contact cooling and suction operational, but with the laser diodes off during the treatment. Patients were evaluated by an independent physician observer. There was an 83% improvement in cellulite, with less dimpling, improved skin tone, and smoothness on the laser-treated side compared to an average 17% improvement on the non-laser-treated side, showing TriActive significantly improves clinical outcomes. Improvements remained for 1 month after treatment. Further study and investigation are required, as the exact mechanism of improvement is not fully understood.

Treatment protocol

Treatments of the body consist of an intensive phase of 12–15 treatment sessions that last 30 min and are scheduled two to three times per week followed up by a maintenance phase. This consists of one to two treatments per month. Any area treated should be clean and free of any lotions or sunscreens. The patient is placed in a prone position. A transverse motion should be carried out from the distal thigh to the proximal thigh and followed by a longitudinal motion, first on the thigh (starting at the distal part) and then on the lower leg (starting from the final part) for two or three passes. Transverse and linear movements on buttocks must also be performed. Treatment takes 25–30 min. Ten to 15 treatments twice a week are recommended (Figure 6.9). Goldman *et al.* [17] evaluated the TriActive device in 11 female patients, all of whom had cellulite on the thighs and/or hips. The group average age was 37.2, an average BMI of 22.76, and average starting body fat percentage of 21.67, measured by electrical impedance. Treatment ran twice weekly using the TriActive device on the lower body, hips, and thighs. Measurements and photos were taken at treatments 5 and 10. A baseline comparison was made to determine if there were any changes in subject BMI or limb circumference. All patients (100%) exhibited observable improvement in cellulite after 10 treatments, with average improvement obtaining a rating of "moderate." There were no reported side effects. Average hip circumference attained a reduction of 1.21 cm, and

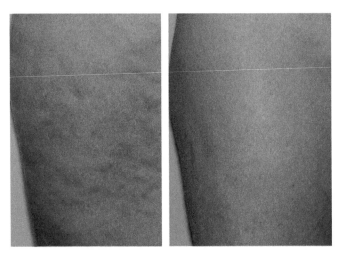

Figure 6.9 TriActive clinical results. Before and after 10 treatments with TriActive.

average thigh reduction was 0.83 cm. No significant change in BMI or body fat percentage was noted in any patient throughout the treatment. This suggests that improvement in cellulite was due to the action of the TriActive device and not changes in other factors. It also suggests that the TriActive device provides localized treatment without effects on any aspect of the body.

VelaSmooth and VelaShape

VelaSmooth (Syneron Medical Ltd., Israel) and VelaShape (Syneron; Figure 6.10) both use Electro-Optical Synergy (ELOS) technology and mechanical manipulation of the skin and fat layer to non-invasively improve the appearance of

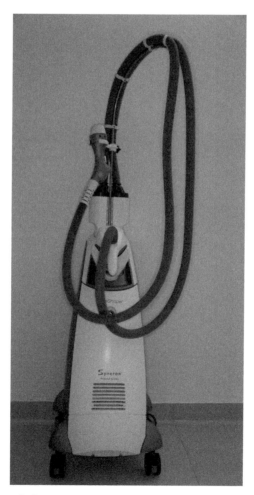

Figure 6.10 VelaShape platform.

cellulite. ELOS is a combination of bipolar RF and optical energies. The rationale of combining the two types of energy is that the RF energy reduces the amount of optical energy needed to achieve a therapeutic effect. Since RF energy does not heat the epidermis, the likelihood of adverse effects such as scarring and skin pigmentation is reduced [18].

There has been improved microcirculation that is affected by the vasodilatory effects and enhanced lymphatic drainage of the negative pressure mechanical massage of this system [18]. Simultaneously, neocollagenesis, collagen contraction, and controlled tissue inflammation are induced by heating tissue by RF and optical energy [19–20]. Since RF is not chromophore targeting, its energy is delivered to penetrate deeper layers of skin tissue without affecting adjacent tissue. The ELOS technology combines these two energy forms, thereby the amount of delivered light energy that is administered to an individual is reduced as compared to the levels at which each alone would have been delivered. This reduces the likelihood of adverse events such as skin pigmentation and scarring.

Mechanism of action

The VelaSmooth provides 20 W of infrared power, 20 W of RF power, 1 MHz RF frequency, and 150 mbar of vacuum suction in 100–300-ms pulses, all delivered directly to the skin through a handheld applicator. Its infrared (IR) light spectrum is 680–1500 nm, and the treated area is 40 mm × 40 mm. The vacuum suction prepares the skin to receive RF energy that penetrates 10 mm [18, 21]. The vacuum suction improves circulation and reduces dimpling by loosening connective tissue around the fat deposits, whereas the IR and RF energies, by heating the skin, enhance the rolling action of the massage unit. Both tissue bulk and dimpling are thus lessened by the massage-induced increase in lymphatic drainage [22]. Analogous to VelaSmooth, the VelaShape device delivers bipolar RF energy, IR light energy, and vacuum suction pulses to the skin surface with a handheld applicator. RF energy penetrates 2–20 mm, whereas IR energy penetrates up to 3 mm beneath the skin. RF power is available at 50 W rather than 20 W (as in VelaSmooth), and the vacuum pattern is modified. With these alterations, treatment duration is shortened approximately 30%, and fewer treatments [4–6] are required to achieve clinical benefit. In addition, the VelaShape platform is available with the VContour applicator. This applicator is smaller and designed for harder to reach areas such as the arms and neck.

It is suggested that heat energy formed by the two energy sources increases the dissociation of oxygen from oxyhemoglobin and its diffusion to adipose tissue. The increase in available oxygen may facilitate an increase in fat metabolism [21]. However, further investigation and support of clinical proof are required to prove this theory. The mechanical massage manipulation of the skin assists in improving circulation and fibrous connective tissue similarly to the mechanism described for TriActive technology earlier in this chapter.

In a pilot study by Wanitphakdeedecha and Manuskiatti [23], they suggested that VelaSmooth treatment improves the bumpiness and dimpling of cellulite. This bumpiness is reduced when the RF current heats adipose tissue at 5–10 mm depths, causing lipolysis and fat chamber shrinkage. As the rollers knead the skin, there is enhanced delivery of RF. The heat also improves peripheral circulation and diffusion of molecules in the treated tissue, thus increasing fat metabolism. The repeated kneading of the skin between the rollers ruptures the sequestered fat cells and temporarily stretches the vertical septa and connective tissue, thereby improving the dimpling.

Treatment protocol

The duration of a typical protocol is about 30–45 min for both VelaSmooth and VelaShape. Patients are well hydrated with greater than 8 ounces of water up to 1 h before treatment. A conductive lotion provided by the manufacturer is applied to further hydrate the skin, and using a handheld applicator, treatment is delivered with four to six passes. The headpiece must be moved back and forth several times over the treatment area. Energy levels are continually adjusted to patient's comfort and tolerance. Gentle but firm pressure is applied to ensure adequate contact of the headpiece to the skin. Endpoints to treatment include erythema and a warm sensation noted by the patient in treated areas that are transient and should disappear within 2 h. Some temporary bruising may been seen after the first several treatments. Hydrate treated area after treatment. Hot baths and showers are avoided for 24 h. The treatment plan requires targeted areas to be treated twice weekly for 4 weeks and then switch to monthly (or less frequently) after that for maintenance.

Sadick and Mulholland [21] conducted the largest study evaluating the effi-cacy of VelaSmooth on 35 patients. This study evaluated the efficacy by observing changes in the circumference of the thighs and estimating improvement (percentage) from photographs taken before and after treatment. Energy levels were dependent on patient tolerance and comfort and were increased with continued treatments. Patients were treated until the appearance of erythema (5–10 min).

It was noted that all patients achieved some level of improvement in cel-lulite appearance and skin smoothing as judged by comparing pretreatment and post-treatment photographs (Figures 6.11 and 6.12). Physician-rated improve-ment was very good to excellent in 23% of patients, good in 35%, and mild in the remaining 42%. The average improvement in cellulite appearance was 40% as judged by a blinded dermatologist. No evidence of structural damage, either epithelial or mesenchymal, was seen on histological analyses of skin biopsy

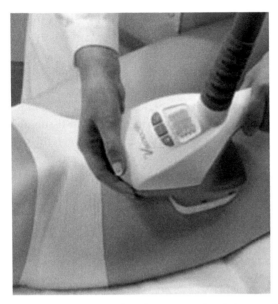

Figure 6.11 Treatment with VelaSmooth – found picture on Google image. (Source: Syneron Medical, Irvine, CA. Reproduced with permission of Syneron Medical.)

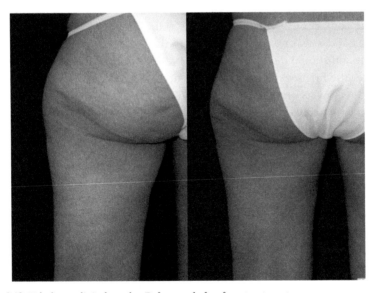

Figure 6.12 Velashape clinical results. Before and after four treatments.

specimens of the lateral thighs taken from three patients before treatment, after two treatments, and after eight treatments.

This initial study was followed up by several other studies conducted, including that of Wanitphakdeedecha and Manuskiatti [23]. They were the first to report cellulite improvement 1 year after a series of treatments with the VelaSmooth and for both the thigh and abdomen. For the thighs, mean circumference reductions were 6.23% immediately after the final treatment, 6.26% 4 weeks later, and 5.50% 1 year later. Mean reductions for the abdomens were 6.32%, 4.04%, and 4.64%, respectively. These results suggest that most of the circumferential reductions are maintained for at least 1 year after the final of eight to nine treatments at two per week.

Romero *et al.* [24] assessed the improvement before and after treatment at several time points by biopsy. Skin biopsy specimens were taken from the buttocks of six of 10 patients before treatment, 2 h after the first treatment, and 2 months after the final of 12 treatments. Results of biopsies taken after the final treatment showed improved epidermal and dermal morphology because of tightened dermal collagen and improved organization of epidermal cells compared to the baseline samples. Specimens taken 2 h after the initial treatment showed dermal fibers aligned with the dermal–epidermal junction, contraction of the papillary dermis, and adipocytes moved close to one another compared to baseline samples (Figure 6.13). This was suggested to be histological changes

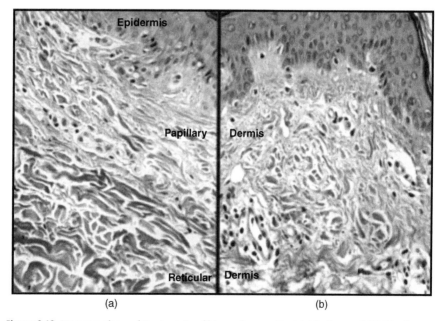

(a)   (b)

Figure 6.13 Hemotoxylin and Eosin stain of biopsy from patient (a) before and (b) 1 h after treatment with VelaShape. Contraction of the papillary dermis is seen, as well as decrease in interfibrillary spaces less fragmentation of collagen fibers.

possibly because of microinflammatory stimuli produced in the treated tissue and subsequent standard tissue repair.

Goldman *et al.* [25] compared the efficacy of treatment of cellulite with the previously described TriActive versus VelaSmooth. Patients were treated twice weekly for 6 weeks with VelaSmooth or TriActive. It was noted that there was a 28% versus a 30% improvement rate, respectively, in the upper thigh circumference measurements, whereas 56% versus a 37% improvement rate was observed, respectively, in lower thigh circumference measurements. Statistical difference of these results was $p > 0.05$. The incidence and extent of bruising were higher for VelaSmooth than for TriActive, which may be attributed to higher mechanical manipulation.

SmoothShapes

SmoothShapes (Eleme Medical, Merrimack NH; Figure 6.14) is a dual energy laser device combining vacuum-assisted mechanical massage capability to stimulate lymphatic and subcutaneous blood flow, new collagen deposition, firming and toning of the skin, and subjective clinical benefits. The dual laser combination employed is a combination of 915-nm near-infrared laser and 650-nm red light from laser diodes.

One of the first studies conducted on SmoothShapes by Neira *et al.* [26] that evaluated the exposure of adipose samples collected from lipectomy to 635-nm wavelengths light from a 10-mW diode laser produced near total emptying of fat from these cells. The authors suggested that this occurrence was due to the transitory pores in the membranes of adipocytes. In addition, they observed that these changes did not cause destruction of adipocytes or other interstitial structures. SmoothShapes added the 915-nm wavelength platform because it can penetrate relatively deep into the skin and has a preferential absorption by lipids. This was established by Anderson *et al.* [27] who showed that four infrared wavelength bands – 915, 1205, 1715, and 2305 nm – have about 50% more absorption in lipid-rich tissue than in aqueous tissue. The combination of 650-nm wavelength for its adipocyte membrane pore-inducing properties and the infrared 915-nm wavelength for its lipid-liquefying properties creates a dual-band light source capable of positively affecting skin adipose tissue. Augmenting this distinct light duo with suction (vacuum) and mechanical massage produces a new therapeutic process called photomotology.

Mechanism of action

The therapeutic effect of low level light therapy has been well supported by numerous studies [28–30]; yet there are questions about how the light works

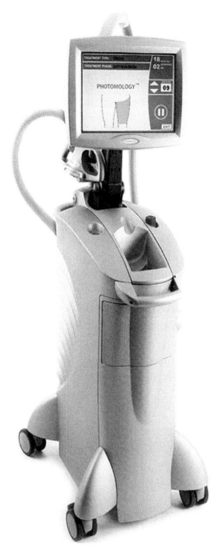

Figure 6.14 SmoothShapes platform. (Source: Cynosure, Westford, MA. Reproduced with permission of Cynosure.)

at the cellular, tissue, and organ levels and what the optimal parameters for the most effective therapeutic effects are. Absorption of monochromatic visible and near-infrared light at the cellular level by components of the cellular respiratory chain is a significant aspect of this understanding [31, 32]. The principal unit within the cell controlling the response to light therapy is the mitochondria. Its involvement of respiratory and ion-transporting activity of the cell produces primary, secondary, and tertiary effects, which collectively enhance tissue repair and produce symptom relief.

This primary effect in cells is referred to as photoreception, which occurs through direct interaction of photons with cytochromes. Cell proliferation is considered the secondary effect in which protein synthesis, growth factor secretion, myfibroblast contraction, and so on occur in the same cells as the primary and can be initiated by light as well as other stimuli. Tertiary effects include tissue repair and wound healing. They are indirect responses of distant cells to photon-induced changes in other cells. These effects are least predictable because they are influenced by cellular as well as environmental factors.

Treatment protocol

The following protocol is designed for a total of eight sessions with SmoothShapes with 20 min per treatment area. The area to be treated is cleansed free of lotions/crèmes. Demarcate the treatment area with a surgical pen; this area is usually defined as approximately 8 inches × 10 inches. The time and treatment area are selected from the menu of the device. Turn on the vacuum button on top of the headpiece and select vacuum grade (low, medium, or high). Activate laser via foot petal. Use inferomedial to superolateral sweeping motion while maintaining firm and even pressure (Figure 6.15). Never sweep headpiece inferiorly down the limb/buttock. Treat until even erythema is the endpoint. It is advised to hydrate the skin after treatment and to avoid hot baths/showers for 24 h after procedure.

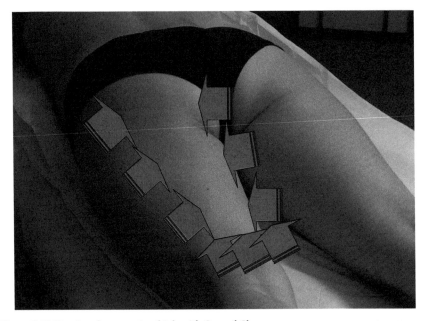

Figure 6.15 Treating the posterior thigh with SmoothShapes.

Lach [33] noted in a study that investigated the efficacy and safety of photomotology by comparing treatment of low level dual-wavelength laser energy and massage with massage alone for the reduction of subcutaneous fat. The fat pad thickness in the treated thighs was objectively assessed by MRI images and evaluated by a blinded radiologist. By quantifiably assessing the measurements using MRI, the fat thickness decreased by $1.19\,cm^2$ (mean) for the laser-massage-treated thigh and increased by $3.82\,cm^2$ (mean) for the leg treated by massage alone. The difference in the changeover time between the laser-massage-treated leg and massage-alone-treated leg was statistically significant ($p < 0.001$). Adverse side reactions to treatment were not seen, and 80.3% would continue maintenance treatments if available (Figure 6.16).

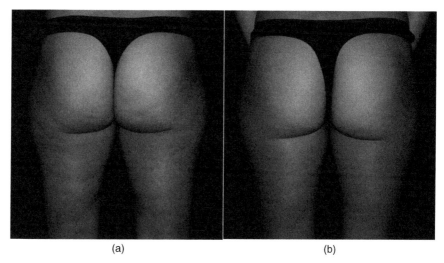

(a)   (b)

Figure 6.16 SmoothShapes clinical result: (a) before and (b) after five treatments with SmoothShapes.

1064 Nd:YAG lasers in cellulite treatment

The use of lasers for adipose tissue removal and tissue tightening has been further investigated with the focus on using a neodymium : yttrium aluminum garnet (Nd:YAG) laser, at a wavelength of 1064 nm. The original principles and technique for this device were initially noted by Blugerman *et al.* using a pulsed 1064-nm Nd:YAG laser [34]. Since then, many investigations have been led related to the use of the 1064-nm Nd:YAG for lipolysis. Laser lipolysis with a pulsed 1064-nm Nd:YAG has been proved a safe and effective method. Badin *et al.* reported its effectiveness in "difficult" cases and so-called "forbidden areas," such as the upper abdomen, upper thigh, and periumbilical region [35].

The Nd:YAG laser targets selected areas of fat for destruction as well as simultaneously tightening the skin [36]. A photoacoustic effect generated by laser selectively destroys the adipocyte membranes, resulting in discharge of cellular contents with minimal risk of tissue charring. The laser also coagulates tissue to promote collagen tightening and hemostasis through the mechanism of photothermolysis. There is a continual evolution in this technology as new applications are being developed to tackle aesthetic issues, including the novel approach to the treatment of cellulite.

Small vessel coagulation and adipocyte rupture were evident after laser irradiation in histological slides. The degree of tumefaction and lysis varied proportionally with the intensity of energy accumulated by the target. The laser-irradiated specimens had adipocyte membrane degeneration, dispersed lipid, and coagulated collagen fibers. Kim and Geronemus [37] evaluated the 1064 Nd:YAG laser for its safety and efficacy. It was noted that there was an energy-dependent relationship, and the amount of volume reduction has been confirmed through mathematical modeling of laser lipolysis [38]. Along with liquefaction of fat, there is a laser–tissue interaction with collagenous and subdermal bands, producing a thermal effect on these tissues, including melting and rupture of the bands. This frees the retracted skin and remodels the collagenous tissue, with clinically evident skin retraction [35].

A study by Goldman *et al.* [39] presents an interesting evaluation to cellulite treatment that combines subdermal Nd:YAG laser lipolysis and autologous fat transplantation (Figure 6.17). In this study, 52 female patients were treated with the pulsed Nd:YAG laser (SmartLipo) that emitted an energy of 6 W, 40 Hz, and 150 mJ/pulse. Laser passes were performed in two planes. In the superficial dermal plane, the action of the laser energy induced neocollagenesis and subsequent skin tightening, whereas in the deeper subcutaneous plane the laser energy was used for overall adipose volume reduction. There was a significant reduction and improvement in cellulite noted at the end of the study. In 84.6%

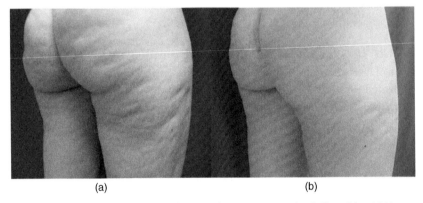

(a)   (b)

Figure 6.17 (a,b) Clinical results of Goldman *et al.* on treatment of cellulite with a 1064-nm Nd:YAG and autologous fat transfer.

of the participants, this resulted in good or excellent outcome with only mild and temporary adverse events. Decreased skin sensibility was a common finding after lipoplasty, but this was found to be transient, lasting several weeks and eventually returning to normal sensibility. The histological findings in this study demonstrated collagen coagulation and degenerative alterations in the fibrous septal connective tissue layer, commonly abnormal in cellulite patients. This procedure is less traumatic than traditional lipoplasty, with patients exhibiting persistent and lasting improvement for over 2 years. The photoacoustic, photomechanical, and photothermal effects of the Nd:YAG laser present a novel and unexploited resource in the treatment of cellulite. Further research is required, and further investigation and establishment of various parameters to fully appreciate the benefits of this technology are necessary.

Use of RF devices for the treatment of cellulite

Radiofrequency devices are heat generating and can lift and tighten dermal tissue, increase the metabolic activity of tissues, and produce a wound healing response that can reduce the appearance of cellulite.

In a study by Alvarez *et al.* [40] using animal models, they showed interesting results of RF treatment on dermal cellularity and collagen formation in guinea pigs. The most relevant changes were seen in the papillary dermis, which underwent expansion as a result of edema and vascular stimulation. These transformations were followed by an increase in cellularity (fibroblasts) and subsequently an increase in collagen, elastin fibers, and mucopolysaccharides. Eventually, all these events lead to increased dermal thickness and collagen content.

Currently, there are two RF devices in the market that are used in the treatment of cellulite and adiposities, the Accent (Alma Lasers, Buffalo Grove IL; Figure 6.18) and Thermage (Thermage, Solta, Hayward, CA; Figure 6.19). Both technologies are U.S. Food and Drug Administration (FDA) approved for the treatment of wrinkles and rhytids. Thermage is a unipolar RF device, whereas the Accent is both unipolar and bipolar RF device. Both of these devices are traditionally used on the face and neck, but buttocks and thighs are more recent additions to the list of applications and show various degrees of efficacy in combating cellulite.

Mechanism of action

Radiofrequency skin tightening is based on the principle of volumetric heating. This heat current is an alternating current, which cycles to and fro at a certain frequency, resulting in ionic agitation in the target tissue. This agitation creates impedance to flow, which generates heat in the tissue, and subsequently

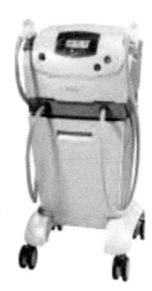

Figure 6.18 Accent laser system. (Source: Alma Lasers, Buffalo Grove, IL. Reproduced with permission of Alma Lasers.)

the tissue tightening effect follows [41]. Subcutaneous fat is considered high impedance tissue and generates large amounts of thermal energy, thus the significant results seen with RF in cellulite control. Unlike light energy, RF current is not scattered by tissue or absorbed by epidermal melanin, therefore patients of all skin types can be treated. RF systems are thought to ameliorate symptoms of cellulite by means of the following three major mechanisms. (i) Dermal tightening of the fibrous septae due to thermal injury affecting the vasculature, which in turn initiates a cascade of inflammatory events, including fibroblastic proliferation and neocollagenesis. (ii) Enhancement of local blood circulation and drainage of fatty acid deposits to the lymphatic system. (iii) Fatty acid dissolution and thermal-induced fat cell apoptosis.

Accent

The accent consists of two headpieces (bipolar and unipolar; Figure 6.20) and an RF generator that operates at a frequency of 40.68 MHz. Both headpieces are used in a continuous sweeping (paint brush) motion while in contact with the skin. The unipolar RF energy penetrates to a depth of about 20 mm, heating the skin tissue and subcutaneous tissue without damage to the tissue surface. The applied RF power for the unipolar headpiece is 100–200 W and 60–100 W for the bipolar headpiece, depending on the clinical application and the treatment area.

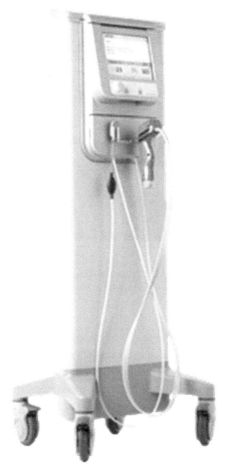

Figure 6.19 Thermage platform. (Source: Solta Medical, San Francisco, CA. Reproduced with permission of Solta Medical.)

Treatment protocol

The patient is advised to remove all jewelry including necklaces, bracelets, and watches. The targeted treatment area marked with grids of approximately 5 cm × 6 cm (15 s exposure time) or 10 cm × 6 cm (30 s exposure time) using a surgical pen. Before the procedure commence, skin should be hydrated with a thin layer of treatment oil to eliminate friction from the movement of the headpiece. The initial treatment parameters should be set according to manufacturer recommendations. In our practice, common cellulite treatment parameters are 150–100 W for a 30-s pass for the unipolar headpiece. For sensitive skin types, power should be reduced by 10–20 W. For oily, acne, sagging, or aging skin, power should be raised 10 W. During each pass, the headpiece is rapidly moved

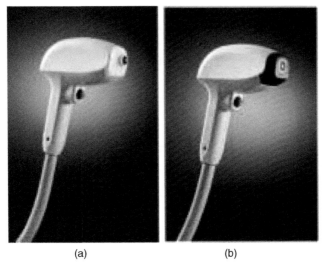

(a)   (b)

Figure 6.20 The unipolar (a) and bipolar (b) handpieces. (Source: Solta Medical, San Francisco, CA. Reproduced with permission of Solta Medical.)

across the skin surface within the grid while applying gentle pressure to maintain uniform contact. The headpiece should be moved in a circular motion covering the entire area within the grid. The epidermal temperature should be monitored throughout the procedure, with a laser thermometer immediately before and after each pass. After reaching the therapeutic threshold of approximately 41°C, the maintenance phase of the treatment can commence. In this case, the energy level and time exposure are reduced 10–15%, and about three additional passes are administered.

A study performed by Goldberg *et al.* [42] used the Accent device for cellulite treatment. Their study included patients with higher grade cellulite of the upper thighs. They were treated every other week for a total of six treatments. Results obtained 6 months after last treatment showed an average 2.45 cm reduction in thigh circumference with minimal side effects, and no changes in serum lipid abnormalities were seen. They attributed the long-lasting effects of this platform to the formation of dermal fibrosis in the upper dermis and increased contraction between the dermis and camper's fascia seen on MRI.

Thermage

Thermage is a noninvasive RF device that delivers monopolar RF energy in the form of an electrical current that generates heat through the inherent electrical resistance of dermal and subcutaneous tissue. The device consists of three main components: a generator, a handheld tip, and a cryogen unit. The generator changes the electric field polarity at the tissue interface at a frequency of 6 million times per second. The handheld tip that contains a cooling device is applied to the skin and protects the epidermis with precooling, parallel cooling, and post-cooling. The headpiece has sensors which monitor temperature and pressure. The depth of heating with this device depends on tip size and geometry. Thermage currently has two tips that are used in the treatment of cellulite, including the deep tissue body tip and the cellulite tip (Figure 6.21). Both tips are able to penetrate depths of about 4.3 mm into the dermis.

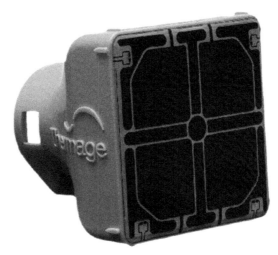

Figure 6.21 Thermage body and cellulite treatment 16.0 body tip. (Source: Solta Medical, San Francisco, CA. Reproduced with permission of Solta Medical.)

Treatment protocol

Problem areas are circled while the patient is standing up. Vectors are drawn in the direction of desired tissue contraction. Apply the 3.0 cm² marking paper to the entire area to be treated. These grid markings should now be visible on the skin. The target area should be completely dry. An initial treatment level setting is selected, which is at the low end of the recommended range (recommended ranges are between 371.5 and 375.0 based on experience during clinical evaluations). A generous amount of coupling fluid is applied to the area to be treated. Gage the setting based on the patient's heat sensation feedback. Preposition skin during treatment. Always pull in the direction of desired skin placement. Perform the first pass across the entire grid (Figure 6.22). During each pulse, be sure to keep the treatment tip perpendicular to the skin ensuring full tip to skin contact and regularly apply coupling fluid. Treatment should be covered in the distal to proximal direction. Treat in medial to lateral direction. At

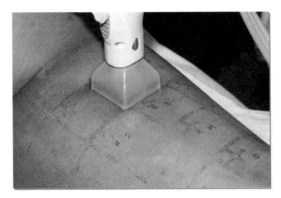

Figure 6.22 Upper thigh treatment with Thermage.

least two to six staggered passes along the entire grid are recommended. Treat to a visible and/or palpable clinical endpoint. Follow-up evaluations are recommended immediately after the treatment and at 3 and 6 months.

Other laser devices for the treatment of cellulite

Two fairly new devices have emerged in the European market, finding a significant level of popularity and drawing curiosity of the North American aesthetics field. It is just a matter of time that both are approved by the FDA and become part of the repertoire of cellulite combating treatments in the United States.

The UltraShape Contour I System (CE 0344; UltraShape Ltd., Yoqneam, Israel; Figure 6.23) is a noninvasive system which by using focused ultrasound selectively disrupts adipocytes by applying thermal or mechanical effects. The system emits focused ultrasound waves to deliver concentrated energy into a focal volume at a precise depth in the subcutaneous tissue. This system was designed to use mechanical (nonthermal) energy to disrupt fat cells and without damaging neighboring structures (skin, blood, and lymph vessels, muscles, and nerves) because of their differential susceptibility to mechanical stresses induced by the ultrasound [43].

One of the first studies conducted on this technology was by Morena-Morago *et al.* in which the efficacy and safety were assessed with a group of 30 healthy patients all treated in the areas of abdomen, inner and outer thighs, flanks, inner knees, and breasts (male patients only). Results showed a significant reduction in subcutaneous fat thickness within those treated areas. The mean reduction in subcutaneous fat thickness after three treatments was 2.28 ± 0.80 cm. Circumference was reduced by a mean of 3.95 ± 1.99 cm. Despite these significant results, it is important to note that this is a technology that requires extensive investigation, in which long-term effects of cellulite treatment should be assessed, especially,

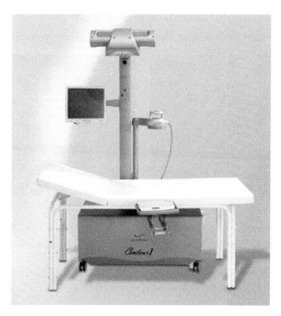

Figure 6.23 Ultrashape device. (Source: Syneron Medical, Irvine, CA. Reproduced with permission of Syneron Medical.)

considerations into the actual effect this device may have on the structure and framework of cellulite.

Utilization of Extracorporeal Pulse Activation Technology (EPAT; Figure 6.24) is another novel approach to cellulite treatment, which has been in use in the European market but has not yet made its way to the United States. High energy acoustic waves are introduced to the targeted areas for cellulite treatment in the form of high frequency oscillation. These pulse waves promote skin

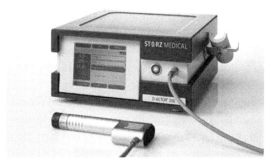

Figure 6.24 EPAT device. (Source: Storz Medical, Tägerwilen, Switzerland. Reproduced with permission of Storz Medical/.)

Clinical evaluation of EPAT

Dermascan (cortex) image of a 54-year-old patient with cellulite

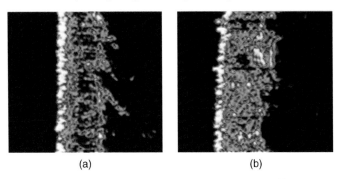

(a)   (b)

Figure 6.25 Collagenometry. Dermascan (Cortex) image of a 54-year-old patient with cellulite. (a) Before EPAT. The dermis/subcutis transitions appear as a very discontinuous irregular line; the black structures are fat cells and lymphatic fluid. (b) After EPAT. The skin structure has become measurably more compact; the zero-echo spaces (black) have reduced further. (Source: Christ C. *et al.* [44]. Reproduced with permission of SAGE.)

tightening by stimulating adipocyte destruction and promoting circulation and lymphatic drainage.

An efficacy study by Christ *et al.* [44] demonstrated that skin elasticity values gradually improved over the course of EPAT therapy and exhibited a 73% increase at the end of therapy. At 3- and 6-month follow-ups, skin elasticity had even improved by 95% and 105%, respectively. Side effects included minor pain for three patients during therapy and slight skin reddening. In the same study, attempting to understand EPAT, Christ *et al.* used collagenometry analyzing the microstructure of cellulite after treatment. The ultrasound evaluation demonstrated increased density and firmness in the network of collagen/elastic fibers in the dermis and subcutis. Treatment was most effective in older patients with a long history of cellulite (Figure 6.25). Further studies are required to better understand this technology and further evaluate its effect on the cellulite structure. Optimal parameters and application of energy should also be further assessed, particularly parameters based on cellulite grades for significant results.

Laser light in the form of far infrared can be used to selectively target fat on the basis of the principles of photothermolysis. Although no devices are available in this format, it was noted by Anderson *et al.* [27] that the 1210- and 1720-nm wavelengths are able to selectively heat adipose tissue. Possible selective laser irradiation of fat at these wavelengths may be another avenue to consider in the future of evolution of technology for the treatment of cellulite.

A recent investigation by O'Dey *et al.* [45] showed fatty tissue ablation using high powered diode laser using fat cells harvested from the anteromedial thigh, *in vitro*. O'Dey claims the 940-nm wavelength successfully increased absorption of both fatty acids and water while maintaining a penetration depth of several millimeters. It was noted that water in the connective tissue septae might be responsible for some of the side effects such as carbonization and enhanced collateral damage leading to vaporization of fat cells. Despite the early stages of these clinical outcomes, there is motivation for further investigation with this technology for cellulite treatment.

Conclusion

Cellulite is a multifactorial condition that represents the most widespread and most complained about aesthetic issue among women. Exhibiting itself as a modification in skin topography, cellulite is evident by skin dimpling and nodularity that occur mainly in women in the pelvic region, lower limbs, and abdomen as a result of the herniation of subcutaneous fat [46] within fibrous connective tissue, leading to a padded or orange-peel appearance. There have been recent advancements in the area of cellulite pathophysiology with several theories that have attracted the attention of scientists with evidence linked to connective tissue alteration and sexually dimorphic skin architecture. A variety of treatment modalities and new technologies continues to evolve to treat the growing concern of cellulite (Table 6.3). Patient demand for less invasive technologies with decreased downtime has led toward the development and application of laser and light sources for the treatment of cellulite. As understanding grows of these modalities, results are variable, and realistic clinical outcomes must be understood by patients. Thermolysis and initiation of collagen remodeling and wound healing response are the basic principles behind these innovative technologies. This heat-induced sequence of events holds a lot of promise in combating cellulite and improving the microcirculation of affected areas. Essentially, the ultimate success lies in the understanding of the early stages of cellulite pathophysiology and fully using optimal treatment parameters to yield tremendous success and further enhance the evolution of cellulite technology.

Table 6.3 Overview of technologies.

Method	Noninvasive	Pain during Tx	Adverse events
VelaShape	Yes	Mild or none	Bruising, erythema, edema
SmoothShapes	Yes	No	Bruising, erythema, edema
Thermage RF	Yes	Mild or none	Rare cutaneous burn due to not enough coupling gel
Accent RF	Yes	No	Blisters, ecchymosis
UltraShape	Yes	No	Bruising, erythema, edema
EPAT	Yes	No	Erythema, edema

References

1 Pierard, G.E. *et al.* (2000) Cellulite: from standing fat herniation to hypodermal stretch marks. *American Journal of Dermatopathology*, **22**, 34–37.

2 Khan, M.H. *et al.* (2010) Treatment of cellulite: Part I. Pathophysiology. *Journal of the American Academy of Dermatology*, **62** (**3**), 361–370.

3 Nurberger, F. & Muller, G. (1978) So-called cellulite: an invented disease. *Journal of Dermatologic Surgery and Oncology*, **4**, 221–229.

4 Querleux *et al.* (2002) Anatomy and physiology of subcutaneous adipose tissue by in vivo MRI and spectroscopy: relationship with sex and presence of cellulite. *Skin Research and Technology*, **8**, 118–124.

5 Curri, S.B. (1976) Aspects morpho-histochimiques et biochimiques du tissue adipeux dans la dermohypodermose cellulitique. *Journal of Medical Esthetics*, **5**, 183.

6 Rossi, A. & Vergnanini, A. (2000) Cellulite: a review. *Journal of the European Academy of Dermatology and Venereology*, **14**, 251–262.

7 Hexsel, D.M. (2001) Body repair. In: Parish, L.C., *et al* (eds), *Women's Dermatology*. Nova Iorque Parthenon Publishing, New York pp. 586–595.

8 Avram, M.A. (2004) Cellulite: a review of its physiology and treatment. *Journal of Cosmetic and Laser Therapy*, **6**, 181–185.

9 Kulick, M. (2006) Evaluation of the combination of radiofrequency, infrared energy, and mechanical rollers with suction to improve surface irregularitites (cellulite) in limited treatment area. *Journal of Cosmetic and Laser Therapy*, **8**, 180–195.

10 Schindl, A. *et al.* (1998) Low-intensity laser irradiation improves skin circulation in patients with diabetic microangiopathy. *Diabetes Care*, **21**, 580–584.

11 Adcock, D. *et al.* (2001) Analysis of the effects of deep mechanical massage in the porcine model. *Plastic and Reconstructive Surgery*, **108**, 233–240.

12 Tanabe, Y. *et al.* (2004) Inhibition of adipocyte differentiation by mechanical stretching through ERK-mediated downregulation of PPARgamma2. *Journal of Cell Science*, **117**, 3605–3614.

13 Berman, D. & Goldberg, A. (1998) Regional differences in adrenergic binding and fat cell lipolysis in obese, post-menopausal women. *Metabolism*, **47**, 467–473.

14 Zerbinati, N., Vergani, R. & Beltrami, B. (2003) *The TriActive System: a Simple and Efficacious Way of Combating Cellulite*. Cynosure, MA.

15 Orringer, J.S. *et al.* (2008) Molecular effects of photodynamic therapy for photoaging. *Archives of Dermatology*, **144**, 1296–1302.

16 Frew, K. & Katz, B. (2003) The efficacy of a diode laser with contact cooling and suction (TriActive System) in the treatment of cellulite. *Presented at the 13th Congress of the European Academy of Dermatology and Venerology*.

17 Goldman, M. & Pabby, A. (2006) Use of TriActive in the treatment of cellulite. In: Goldman, M., Bacci, P., Leibaschoff, G., Hexsel, D. & Angelini, F. (eds), *Cellulite Pathology and Treatment* Informa Healthcare, New York.

18 Sadick, N. & Magro, C. (2007) A study evaluating the safety and efficacy of the VelaSmooth system in the treatment of cellulite. *Journal of Cosmetic and Laser Therapy*, **9**, 15–20.

19 Hantash, B. *et al.* (2009) Bipolar fractional radiofrequency treatment induced neoelastogenesis and neocollagenesis. *Lasers in Surgery and Medicine*, **41**, 1–9.

20 Kuo, T. *et al.* (1998) Collagen thermal damage and collagen synthesis after cutaneous laer resurfacing. *Lasers in Surgery and Medicine*, **23**, 66–71.

21 Sadick, N. & Mulholland, R. (2004) A prospective clinical study to evaluate the efficacy and safety of cellulite treatment using the combination of optical and RF energies for subcutaneous tissue heating. *Journal of Cosmetic and Laser Therapy*, **6**, 187–190.

22 Alster, T. & Tehrani, M. (2006) Treatment of cellulite with optical devices: an overview with practical considerations. *Lasers in Surgery and Medicine*, **38**, 727–730.

23 Wanitphakdeedecha, R. & Manuskiatti, W. (2006) Treatment of cellulite with bipolar radiofrequency, infrared heat, and pulsatile suction device: a pilot study. *Journal of Cosmetic Dermatology*, **5**, 284–288.

24 Romero, C. *et al.* (2008) Effects of cellulite treatment with RF, IR light, mechanical massage and suction treating one buttock with the contralateral as a control. *Journal of Cosmetic and Laser Therapy*, **10**, 193–201.

25 Nootheti, P.K., Magpantay, A., Yosowitz, G., Calderon, S. & Goldman, M. (2006) A single center, randomized, comparative prospective clinical study to determine the efficacy of the VelaSmooth system versus the TriActive system for the treatment of cellulite. *Lasers in Surgery and Medicine*, **38**, 908–912.

26 Neira, R. *et al.* (2002) Fat liquefaction: effect of low-level laser energy on adipose tissue. *Plastic and Reconstructive Surgery*, **100**, 912–922.

27 Anderson, R.R. *et al.* (2006) Selective photothermolysis of lipid rick tissues: a free electron laser study. *Lasers in Surgery and Medicine*, **38**, 913–919.

28 Gupta, A.K. *et al.* (1998) The use of low energy photon therapy in venous leg ulcers: a double blind, placebo-controlled study. *Dermatologic Surgery*, **24**, 1383–1386.

29 Hamblin, M.R. *et al.* (2006) Mechanisms of low level light therapy. In: Hamblin, M.R., Waynant, R.W. & Anders, J. (eds), *Mechanism of Low Level Light Therapy, Proceedings of SPIE*. Vol. **6140001**, pp. 1–12.

30 Hawkins, D. *et al.* (2005) Low level laser therapy (LLLT) as an effective therapeutic modality for delayed wound healing. *Annals of the New York Academy of Sciences*, **1056**, 486–493.

31 Enwemeka, C.S. (2001) Attenuation and penetration of visible 632 and invisible 904 infra-red light in soft tissue. *Laser Therapy*, **13**, 95–101.

32 Grimblatov, V. *et al.* (2006) Spectral dosimetry in low light therapy. In: Hamblin, M.R., Waynant, R.W. & Anders, J. (eds), *Mechanism of Low Level Light Therapy, Proceedings of SPIE*. Vol. **6140001**, pp. 1–12.

33 Lach, E. (2008) Reduction of subcutaneous fat and improvement in cellulite appearance by dual-wavelength, low-level laser energy combined with vacuum and massage. *Journal of Cosmetic and Laser Therapy*, **10**, 202–209.

34 Blugerman, G.E. & Schavelzon, D. (2000) Laserlipolisis: la modelacion corporal def neuvo milenio. In: *Studo Grafico*. Buenos Aires, Argentina.

35 Badin, A., Moraes, L., Gondek, L. *et al.* (2002) Laser lipolysis: flaccidity under control. *Aesthetic Plastic Surgery*, **26**, 335–339.

36 Khan, M.H. *et al.* (2010) Treatment of cellulite: Part II. Advances and Controversies. *Journal of the American Academy of Dermatology*, **62** (**3**), 72–84.

37 Kim, K. & Geroneum, R.G. (2006) Laser lipolysis using a novel 1064 nm neodymium: yttrium-aluminum-garnet laser. *Dermatologic Surgery*, **32**, 246–253.

38 Mordon, S.R., Wassmer, B., Reynaud, J.P. & Zemmouri, J. (2008) Mathematical modeling of laser lipolysis. *Biomedical Engineering Online*, **29**, 7–10.

39 Goldman *et al.* (2008) Cellulite: a new treatment approach combining subdermal Nd:YAG laser lioplysis and autologous fat transplantation. *Aesthetic Surgery Journal*, **28**, 656–662.

40 Alvarez, N. *et al.* (2008) The effects of radiofrequency on skin: an experimental study. *Lasers in Surgery and Medicine*, **40**, 76–82.

41 Emilia del Pino, M. *et al.* (2006) Effect of controlled volumetric tissue heating with radiofrequency on cellulite and the subcutaneous tissue of the buttocks and thighs. *Journal of Drugs and Dermatology*, **5**, 714–722.

42 Goldberg *et al.* (2008) Clinical, laboratory, and MRI analysis of cellulite treatment with a unipolar radiofrequency device. *Journal of Dermatologic Surgery*, **34**, 204–209.

43 Moreno-Moraga, J. *et al.* (2007) Body contouring by non-invasive transdermal focused ultra-sound. *Lasers in Surgery and Medicine*, **39**, 315–323.

44 Christ, C. *et al.* (2008) Improvement in skin elasticity in the treatment of cellulite and con-nective tissue weakness by means of extracorporeal pulse activation therapy. *Aesthetic Surgery Journal*, 538–544.

45 O'Dey *et al.* (2008) Ablative targeting of fatty-tissue using a high powered diode laser. *Lasers in Surgery and Medicine*, **40**, 100–105.

46 Draelos, Z.D. & Marenus, K.D. (1997) Cellulite – etiology and purported treatment. *Derma-tologic Surgery*, **23**, 1177–1181.

CHAPTER 7

Cooling for fat

Andrew A. Nelson

Nelson Dermatology, FL, USA
Department of Dermatology, Tufts University School of Medicine, MA, USA

Introduction

Body sculpting and fat removal are some of the most troubling issues faced by patients as they seek to achieve their ideals of beauty. Fat removal is a billion dollar industry, and liposuction continues to remain the most common surgical cosmetic procedure performed in the United States [1]. Over the last decade, patients are increasingly turning to minimally invasive procedures, requiring little, if any, downtime, to achieve their cosmetic goals. The treatment of fat is not different. While liposuction remains the gold standard treatment, it is an invasive procedure requiring at the very least tumescent anesthesia and a recovery period. Furthermore, many patients have localized, relatively small problem areas of excess fat. Many of these patients do not wish to undergo liposuction, and would prefer a noninvasive, minimal downtime procedure. While many differing technologies have been advocated for noninvasive fat removal including radiofrequency, ultrasound, and lasers, these techniques have typically only resulted in modest clinical improvements in the appearance of fat. More recently, a novel technology known as cryolipolysis has been developed. Cryolipolysis has been reported to result in clinically significant improvements in body contour and reductions in fat layer thickness. While the results do not compare to those of liposuction procedures, cryolipolysis represents a breakthrough in the safe, noninvasive treatment of subcutaneous fat via the selective destruction of adipocytes. This technology provides modest, but real reductions in fat layer thickness with minimal downtime, and few side effects.

Cold exposure has long been anecdotally reported to be associated with alterations in adipose tissue. This phenomenon was first reported in young children, when it is referred to as "popsicle panniculitis" [2, 3]. Approximately 24–72 h after cold exposure, such as after sucking on an ice cube, infants were noted to develop firm, erythematous, subcutaneous nodules in the area. A similar clinical entity has also been reported in horseback riders exposed to cold, when it is known as equestrian panniculitis [4]. Histologic study of these conditions reveals that following the cold exposure, inflammation of the dermis and adipose tissue results. Approximately 24 h after cold exposure, a perivascular histiocytic and lymphocytic infiltrate develops at the dermal–subcutaneous junction with spread into the adipose tissue. Over the next several days, the inflammation becomes more denser with additional neutrophils, lymphocytes, histiocytes, and monocytes being recruited to the affected area. Ultimately, adipocyte necrosis can be observed. This inflammation and adipocyte change typically spontaneously resolves over the next several weeks with no long-term damage to the affected area. These clinical observations support the idea that localized cold exposure can be used to selectively target and damage underlying adipose tissue. On the basis of these observances, cryolipolysis was investigated as a potential noninvasive fat removal strategy. The next step was to determine whether these observations could help to develop a novel noninvasive treatment for excess fat.

Cryolipolysis

Preclinical studies
The initial studies of cryolipolysis were conducted in Yucatan pigs. The first article reporting the effects of cryolipolysis actually described three separate preclinical studies. The initial exploratory study consisted of application of a circular copper plate attached to a chiller, thereby maintaining a constant temperature of $-7\,^{\circ}$C. The cold copper plate was applied to the skin of the pig for between 5 and 21 min, and the treated area was followed for 3.5 months following the exposure. The greatest effect was noted on the buttocks, where 40% of the total fat (80% of the superficial fat layer) was removed following the single cryolipolysis treatment [5]. This initial exploratory study documented the potential efficacy of controlled cold exposure in reducing excess fat.

A prototype clinical device (Zeltiq Aesthetics, Pleasanton, CA) was then developed, which employed a thermoelectric cooling element to maintain a variable, constant, preset temperature. The pig tissue was then exposed to cold exposures, ranging between 20 and $-7\,^{\circ}$C for 10 min. The tissue was treated in a flat configuration, where a single plate was applied to the skin, as well as a folded configuration, where the skin was pinched between two treatment plates. This serves to maximize the surface area of treatment as well as to restrict blood flow to the treated area. By restricting blood flow, the cooling of the tissue can be achieved more efficiently.

All sites treated with a temperature less than $-1\,^{\circ}C$ developed fat layer reduction, perivascular inflammation, and panniculitis. Fat damage and removal was significantly greater at lower temperatures and in the folded configuration as this allowed for more effective cooling of the tissue as described earlier. Substantial reductions in fat layer thickness were again observed following cryolipolysis treatments.

Finally, lipid profiles were obtained during the course of this study. In all cases, no significant alteration of the lipid profiles of the animals was noted immediately following the treatment or in the 3-month extended follow-up period. A transient decrease in triglyceride levels was noted immediately following the treatment, although this was attributed by the authors to the animals fasting before general anesthesia, rather than a direct effect of the treatment itself. These initial studies documented the efficacy as well as the safety profile of cryolipolysis.

Proposed mechanism of action

Although the exact mechanism of action has not been fully elucidated, case reports and preclinical studies have helped to establish the most likely explanation for the process of cryolipolysis. As the cooling takes place, the lipids in adipocytes crystallize. Following treatment, it is likely that the first effect after cold exposure is apoptosis or necrosis of the adipocytes. In animal studies, adipocytes cooled to temperatures of -2, 0, and $2\,^{\circ}C$ underwent apoptosis or necrosis; the majority of adipocytes cooled to temperatures less than $7\,^{\circ}C$ also underwent apoptosis or necrosis [6]. Adipocytes cooled to temperatures between 14 and $28\,^{\circ}C$ did not show these effects. Thus, there appears to be a critical temperature below which adipocytes will become necrotic and apoptotic. It is still unclear as to why the adipocytes are more sensitive to cold exposure, and why they appear to be more sensitive than other tissues.

Immediately following the treatment, no significant histologic alterations in the subcutaneous fat layer are observed. However, over the following 1–3 days, an inflammatory infiltrate develops; this is likely in response to adipocyte necrosis and apoptosis. Initially, a localized mixed inflammatory infiltrate composed predominantly of neutrophils and mononuclear cells develops in the subcutaneous layer. The inflammatory infiltrate appears to peak at the 14th day following treatment, and is manifested as a lobular panniculitis consisting of histiocytes, neutrophils, lymphocytes, and other mononuclear cells (Figure 7.1a–c). Between days 14 and 30, the inflammatory panniculitis becomes less dense and phagocytosis of the lipids becomes evident. Macrophages

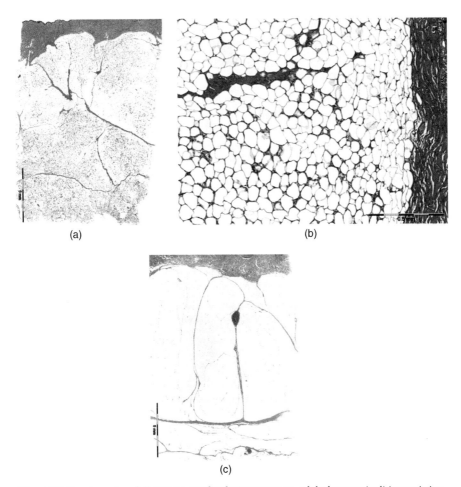

(a)   (b)

(c)

Figure 7.1 Fourteen days following a cryolipolysis treatment, a lobular panniculitis consisting of histiocytes, neutrophils, lymphocytes, and other mononuclear cells peaks (low power shown in (a) and high power shown in (b)). For comparison, an untreated control area is shown in (c). (Source: Dr. Eric Okamoto (Fremont, CA), Drs David Kaufman and Christa Clark (Folsom, CA). Reproduced with permission of Eric Okamoto, David Kaufman, and Christa Clark.)

surround and engulf the dead adipocytes as the body's immune system attempts to eliminate these apoptotic cells. As this process occurs, the average size of the adipocytes decreases, a wider range of adipocyte sizes are observed, and the fibrous septae of the fat layer become widened [7, 8]. During the next 90 days, the inflammatory infiltrate decreases further, the adipocytes are cleared, and the thickness of the subcutaneous fat layer is gradually decreased (Figure 7.2a–c).

The reduction in the subcutaneous fat layer is achieved gradually over at least 90 days following a cryolipolysis treatment. The end result is a decrease

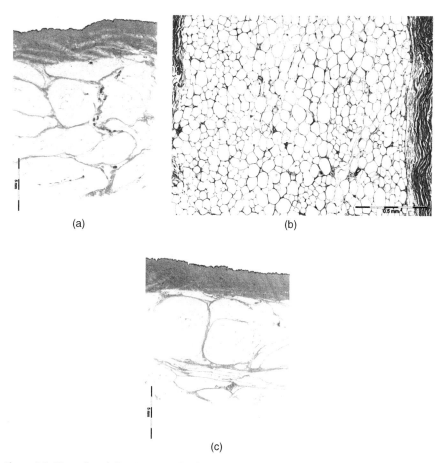

(a)   (b)

(c)

Figure 7.2 Ninty days following a cryolipolysis treatment, the inflammatory infiltrate has
decreased significantly, the adipocytes are clearing, and the thickness of the subcutaneous fat
layer has gradually decreased (low power shown in (a) and high power shown in (b)). For
comparison, an untreated control area is shown in (c). (Source: Dr. Eric Okamoto (Fremont,
CA), Drs David Kaufman and Christa Clark (Folsom, CA). Reproduced with permission of Eric
Okamoto, David Kaufman, and Christa Clark.)

in the size of the lobules of fat cells, which in turn allows the fibrous septae to
constitute a majority of the volume of the subcutaneous tissue. These changes
correspond with the clinical effects seen following cryolipolysis. To date, the exact
mechanism and pathway by which the adipocytes are cleared from the body has
not been fully elucidated. The slow elimination of the fat cells over a prolonged
period of time is likely responsible for the gradual effect of cryolipolysis, as well as
the consistency of lipid levels following treatment. These gradual effects suggest
a safe mechanism of elimination and are likely responsible for the strong safety
profile of cryolipolysis.

Clinical effects of cryolipolysis

CoolSculpting® (Zeltiq Aesthetics, Pleasanton, CA) is the only U.S. Food and Drug Administration (FDA) cleared device for noninvasive fat reduction utilizing cryolipolysis technology. The CoolSculpting device consists of a treatment console with an applicator attached by a cable (Figure 7.3). The treatment area on the patient is covered with a thermal coupling gel sheet to ensure consistent contact and the applicator is attached (Figure 7.4a,b). When applied to the skin, any air pockets should be removed from the gel sheet in order to maximize contact with the skin. A moderate vacuum is created by the device to draw the tissue up in between two cooling plates. This serves to restrict blood flow to the treated tissue, thus making heat extraction easier. A cooling intensity factor (CIF) is selected by the treating physician, which represents the rate of heat flux out of the tissue during the treatment. The selected heat extraction rate (cooling) is modulated by thermoelectric cooling cells and controlled by sensors that monitor the heat flux out of the tissue. Once the applicator is positioned and the CIF is selected by the physician, no further operator intervention is necessary during

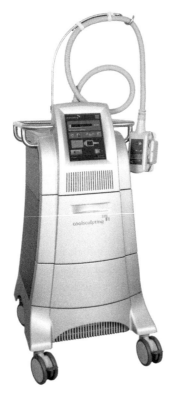

Figure 7.3 The CoolSculpting treatment device. (Source: Zeltiq, Pleasanton, CA. Reproduced with permission of Zeltiq.)

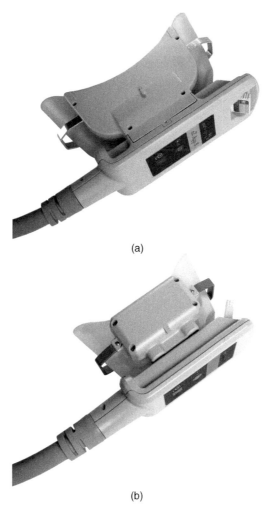

(a)

(b)

Figure 7.4 (a) The CoolSculpting treatment applicator, (b) the applicator with the thermal coupling gel sheet and both cooling plates in place.   (Source: Zeltiq, Pleasanton, CA. Reproduced with permission of Zeltiq.)

the treatment cycle, which can last up to 60 minutes. The patient can alert a physician or nurse via a paging system connected to the device in the event of a question or concern.

At the outset of treatment, some patients experience mild discomfort, especially with larger hand pieces over the abdomen. This discomfort improves greatly at 6–8 min into treatment as the cutaneous nerves begin to numb. Before the completion of the treatment cycle, the treated tissue is automatically massaged by the hand piece for several minutes. Patients often can feel the massage occur. At the termination of treatment, a pager alerts the physician.

Once the cycle is completed, the cooling cycle automatically terminates and the physician releases the vacuum thereby completing the treatment. The treated area is typically erythematous and molded into the shape of the hand piece. It is anesthetic as well. With thawing, the molding disappears within minutes. Depending on the areas to be treated, multiple applications during the same visit can be performed to achieve the treatment goals. After treatment, the treated area is massaged by the operator in order to break up the crystallized adipocytes. This is thought to improve clinical results.

A multicenter, randomized trial demonstrated fat reduction with CoolSculpting in the treatment of the flank (love handles) and back (back fat pads) [9]. Patients in this study were randomized to have one side of the body treated, while the contralateral side served as an untreated control. Clinical efficacy was determined utilizing multiple methods, including digital photography, patient self-assessment, physician assessment, and ultrasound analysis. An interim subgroup analysis of 32 treated patients demonstrated that all of the patients had achieved a clinical improvement, manifested as a visible contour change, 4 months following a single cryolipolysis treatment. Ultrasound analysis demonstrated a reduction in fat layer thickness in all treated patients, with a mean reduction of 22.4% (Figure 7.5). Significantly, the best cosmetic results were achieved in patients with a discrete, modest fat bulge. CoolSculpting was well-tolerated by patients, with no adverse events reported.

Kaminer *et al.* [10] also documented the clinical efficacy of CoolSculpting for the treatment of flank and back fat. A blinded photographic comparison of patients preprocedure and 6 months following a single CoolSculpting procedure was performed on 50 patients. Three physicians, specializing in dermatology, cosmetic surgery, and plastic surgery, analyzed the digital images. In 89% of the cases, the physicians were able to reliably differentiate between the pre- and post-procedure images. A subgroup analysis was then performed on patients who maintained a constant weight during the follow-up period, and the physicians were able to accurately differentiate 92% of the pre- and post-procedure images.

Most recently, CoolSculpting has been studied for potential efficacy in the treatment of abdominal fat. A total of 42 patients were treated with CoolSculpting on symmetric abdominal fat bulges, located to the right and left of the umbilicus [11]. An interim analysis demonstrated that 79% (31 out of 39 subjects) reported clinical improvement in the appearance of their abdominal fat 2–4 months following a single CoolSculpting treatment.

These studies support the clinical efficacy of cryolipolysis and the CoolSculpting device for fat layer reduction. The improvement is limited, but nonetheless real. The data support that the effect seems to be most significant for discrete, localized fat bulges – typically areas that are resistant to improvement with diet and exercise. Patients should be counseled that CoolSculpting will result in a visible, significant contour change that develops gradually in the months following their treatment.

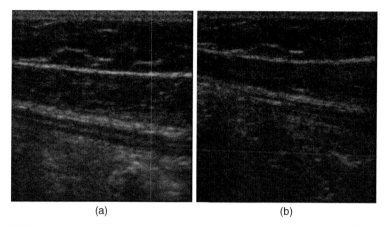

(a)   (b)

Figure 7.5 Ultrasound images reveal a marked reduction in the thickness of the subcutaneous fat layer before (a) and 4 months after (b) following a single CoolSculpting treatment. (Source: Dr. Michael Kaminer, Chestnut Hill, MA. Reproduced with permission of Michael Kaminer.)

Patient selection

The proper selection of patients is essential to a successful cryolipolysis treatment. Cryolipolysis results in a gradual reduction of localized areas of fat following the treatment. It is not a treatment for obesity or weight loss, and should not be used on patients who are seeking large-scale fat removal. Moreover, it will not achieve results comparable to liposuction with one treatment.

The ideal patient for cryolipolysis is a relatively fit patient who has localized, discrete areas of excess fat. Many times these patients have dieted and exercised extensively, but have difficulty in eliminating certain areas of fat accumulation. The most common treatment areas are the flank ("the love handles"), the back ("back fat pads"), and the abdomen ("muffin top") (Figure 7.6). The ideal patient is seeking a quick, noninvasive, minimal downtime procedure to treat these areas of small, localized excess fat. They also understand that the treatment will result in improvement gradually over 2–4 months following the procedure.

For the device to function properly, it must be able to create a vacuum around the treatment area in order to pinch the skin between the two treatment plates. The ideal patient will have a localized area of excess fat that can be pinched and elevated by the physician (Figure 7.7); the treatment area should also fit within the CoolSculpting applicator, or the patient will require multiple treatment applications (Figure 7.8). If the area for which the patient is seeking treatment cannot be pinched and elevated by the physician, then they may not be a good candidate for this procedure. Abdominal girth that results from an accumulation of visceral fat will not be improved with cryolipolysis.

Finally, cryolipolysis is not an alternative to large volume liposuction. Patients, who are obese, or seeking a large volume fat removal should not

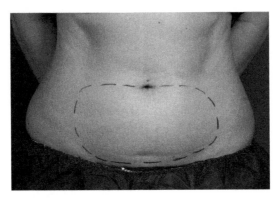

Figure 7.6 Patient with discrete, localized area of excess fat across the abdomen (the "muffin top"). The localized area of excess fat is marked before beginning the treatment. (Source: Zeltiq, Pleasanton, CA. Reproduced with permission of Zeltiq.)

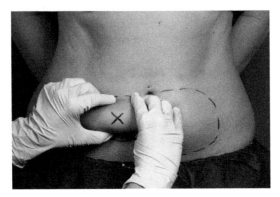

Figure 7.7 The proposed treatment area should be pinched and elevated by the physician. If the area for which the patient is seeking treatment cannot be pinched and elevated by the physician, then they may not be a good candidate for this procedure. (Source: Zeltiq, Pleasanton, CA. Reproduced with permission of Zeltiq.)

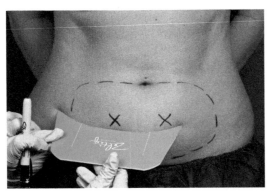

Figure 7.8 The size of the proposed treatment area is then compared with the size of the applicator. In this case, two treatment applications (each marked with an X), will be necessary to adequately treat the abdomen. (Source: Zeltiq, Pleasanton, CA. Reproduced with permission of Zeltiq.)

undergo cryolipolysis. Rather, if a patient is seeking instant, massive fat removal, then they should be most likely to undergo liposuction or bariatric surgery, and should be referred to an appropriate specialist.

Consultation

The consultation is an important opportunity for the physician to assess the patient, their problem areas, their goals and expectations, and their suitability for the procedure. During the consultation, physicians should assess the patient's body type to determine if they are a good candidate for CoolSculpting. They should also assess the patient's desired treatment areas in order to determine the likely efficacy of CoolSculpting, as well as how many treatment applications will be necessary.

The consultation is also a great opportunity for the physician to educate the patient regarding the cryolipolysis procedure, answer their questions, and most importantly, set realistic expectations. It is important to remind patients that the clinical efficacy of CoolSculpting will not develop immediately, but rather will develop gradually in the first few months following the treatment. It is also important to emphasize that results will vary among patients. For some patients, there may be no discernible.

Preoperative procedures/considerations

There are no significant preoperative tests that need to be performed before cryolipolysis. It is helpful to obtain high quality images of the patient before the procedure. The fat sculpting effect of cryolipolysis occurs slowly over several weeks to months following the procedure; as a result, having high quality pre- and post-procedure pictures can be of benefit in assessing the final clinical improvement. We recommend taking pictures from several different angles, and repeating these pictures 3–4 months following the procedure to fully assess the patient's improvement if necessary.

Patients should also be examined to determine the number of applications they will require during their treatment. For instance, if the patient requires both love handles to be treated, this may require two applications (one for each side). Multiple applications increase the length of time necessary for the procedure, and will have an impact on the cost of the procedure. More treatments will result in a more dramatic clinical result for a given area. The patient and physician should discuss and plan appropriately regarding the number of applications necessary to achieve the patient's ultimate treatment goal.

Pearls

- A consultation before treatment is strongly recommended. It is essential to convey to the patient that the procedure provides modest fat layer reduction. In fact, some patients may see less than the modest improvement. Cryolipolysis is not an alternative to liposuction, but rather a more limited means to achieve noninvasive fat reduction. Multiple treatment cycles will produce a more dramatic clinical result.
- Patients should also be advised that in a small percentage of patients, a pain syndrome may follow treatment, beginning 3–4 days after the procedure. It can persist for 2–3 weeks. In rare cases, there may be a paradoxical increase in fat in the treated area.
- While examining the patient, pinch the fat that has to be treated. Some protuberant abdomens are not conducive for the procedure. For example, patients with a great deal of visceral fat will experience no improvement with this treatment because it is only effective for subcutaneous fat. If the subcutaneous fat cannot be adequately pinched, the procedure will not be effective.
- Before treatment, assess for any evidence of hernia. The suction could potentially aggravate such a condition. Caution is advised in any patient with a history of hernia. Similarly, caution is advised when treating over a surgical scar.
- Manual massage after treatment may improve efficacy.
- Treat one area first to assess for efficacy. If it is found to be effective, other areas can be subsequently treated.
- Separate treatments to the same area by 2–3 months in order to maximize the benefit to the patient.
- Spend a few minutes at the outset of the procedure in the room with the patient to assess comfort and answer any questions or concerns.
- Before treatment of small fat accumulations, it is often advisable to attempt to attach the hand piece to the area to determine if there is sufficient fat for the device to operate. This can avoid waste of time for the patient and the physician. With new treatment hand pieces that better conform to the body shape of the patient, this concern has receded. However, if there is insufficient fat, the device will not operate.

Complications: how to avoid them and how to treat them

In clinical studies, cryolipolysis has been proven to be a safe procedure. CoolSculpting is considered to be a noninvasive, no downtime procedure. There are, however, mild immediate effects on the treated area. Most typically, patients will develop erythema of the area immediately following the treatment; this erythema resolves over the next several hours. The area is also cool to touch, and may be slightly firm following the treatment (Figures 7.9–7.11). Bruising of the area can occur, although this is more likely due to the vacuum device rather than the actual fat cooling. These are transient effects and do not require any treatment; rather, the patient should be educated about these temporary effects before undergoing the procedure. Infrequently, patients experience a distinctive pain syndrome beginning 3–4 days following treatment. This is not the same as localized posttreatment tenderness following treatment. Rather, the pain can be "sharp" and "shooting." It can persist for 2–3 weeks, but is self-resolving with no long-term clinical sequelae. Pain medication regimens and reassurance are crucial to provide comfort to the patient during these episodes.

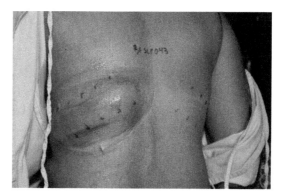

Figure 7.9 Immediately after one CoolSculpting treatment application, the patient's treatment area on the back "the back fat," appears erythematous and swollen. The area is also cool to touch. (Source: Dr. Ivan Rosales-Berber, San Luis Potosi, Mexico. Reproduced with permission of Ivan Rosales-Berber.)

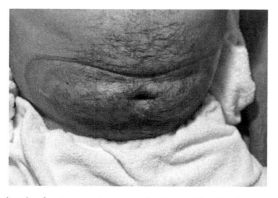

Figure 7.10 Immediately after two treatment applications of CoolSculpting, the patient's abdomen "the muffin top," appears erythematous and swollen. The area is also cool to touch. (Source: Dr. Kathleen Welsh, San Francisco, CA. Reproduced with permission of Kathleen Welsh.)

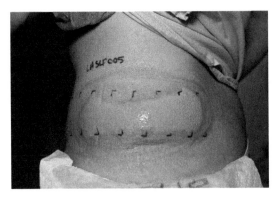

Figure 7.11 Immediately after one CoolSculpting treatment application, the patient's treatment area on the flank "the love handle," appears erythematous and swollen. The area is also cool to touch. (Source: Dr. Ivan Rosales-Berber, San Luis Potosi, Mexico. Reproduced with permission of Ivan Rosales-Berber.)

Recently, there have been reports of a paradoxical increase of fat in the area of treatment following cryolipolysis [12]. Demographic study of patients experiencing this side effect has not elucidated who is at highest risk. Further, there is an unknown mechanism of action to explain this side effect. Typically, there is a decrease in fat layer thickness at 2–3 months that transforms to an increase in fat in the area of treatment. The area of fat increase correlates to the size and shape of the applicator.

Importantly, in all clinical studies to date, no cases of ulceration, scarring, or permanent pigmentary change have been reported.

Cryolipolysis has also been noted to cause temporary altered sensation in the treated areas. In clinical studies, patients have reported dullness of sensation and numbness in the area. In order to characterize the frequency of this effect, a clinical study of 10 subjects underwent unilateral treatment of one "love handle" with the cryolipolysis while the other untreated side served as a contralateral control [13]. Patients were examined clinically and via ultrasound to assess the improvement in the fat layer, and also underwent a neurologic assessment with a board-certified physician to assess any potential altered neurologic sensation. Following a single treatment with the device, patients achieved a significant improvement in the clinical appearance of their fat, as well as an ultrasound measured thickness of the fat layer, indicating a successful treatment. The majority of patients (24/25 of areas treated, 96%) reported numbness immediately following the procedure, although by 1 week the symptoms were improving and/or resolved. On clinical neurologic examination, six of the nine patients (67%) were noted to have reduced pain and pinprick sensation at 1 week following cryolipolysis. Four subjects were noted to have reduced responses to light touch, which became apparent 1–2 weeks following the treatment and spontaneously resolved over the following 2 weeks. Variable temporary alterations in two-point discrimination and temperature sensation were also observed in a minority of the patients. The mean duration of the altered sensation was 3.6 weeks, with a range of 1–6 weeks. In all cases, the neurologic alterations were temporary and spontaneously resolved with no intervention necessary. Physicians should discuss the possibility of temporary altered sensation with their patients before undergoing cryolipolysis, and reiterate that while this effect may occur, it is transient and will require no treatment.

   Patients may also be concerned about possible systemic side effects of the cryolipolysis. They may also wonder, whether the treated fat goes into their blood or alters their lipid profile. Clinical studies have been performed to characterize any potential effects on the blood lipid profile, and they have documented that cryolipolysis appears to have no significant impact. In the initial preclinical animal studies, no significant changes in the blood lipid or liver profile were observed following multiple cryolipolysis treatments of large body surface areas [14]. Human clinical studies have also shown no significant changes in lipid profiles or liver function tests following cryolipolysis. In a clinical study, 40 patients underwent cryolipolysis treatment to their bilateral love handles; some subjects required two applications to completely treat each love handle, with a maximum of four total applications to complete the treatment [15]. Patients were treated with the CoolSculpting device at a CIF of 42 for 30 min. The patients underwent blood lipid and liver testing at a pretreatment baseline, as well as 1 day and 1, 4, 8, and 12 weeks after the treatment. No significant alterations in liver function values were noted at any time point in the study. Mean cholesterol levels did not significantly change following the treatment. Triglyceride values were noted to increase slightly in the weeks following the cryolipolysis treatment, from a mean of 82.1 to 93.2, although this increase was not statistically significant. A statistically significant decline in high-density lipoprotein (HDL) values did occur following cryolipolysis, particularly in the 1st week following the treatment, but these values returned to baseline by the completion of the study 12 weeks following treatment. As the HDL values remained above the lower limit of the normal range, it is unclear whether this transient decrease would have any clinical significance. Owing to this strong safety profile, there is no requirement to check blood lipid or liver function tests in patients undergoing cryolipolysis treatments.

   Cryolipolysis is a safe and effective method for patients to achieve clinically significant reductions in fat layer thickness. Physicians should counsel their patients on temporary, self-resolving changes to the skin that may occur following treatment such as erythema, bruising, and dulling of sensation in the treatment area. However, patients should be reminded that these side effects are minor, temporary, and self-resolving.

Postoperative care/considerations

In the postoperative period, no significant care is required for the patient. Patients can return to their normal activities. The area may feel cool and slightly firm to the touch. There will also be a localized hypoesthesia in the area of treatment. This will spontaneously resolve and requires no intervention on the patient's part. Patients may develop some mild bruising of the treatment area due to the vacuum effect of the device, and as a result, they may want to avoid aspirin and other nonsteroidal anti-inflammatory drugs (NSAIDs), which could theoretically worsen the bruising. Patients should be instructed not to apply cold compresses to the area following treatment in an effort to diminish the bruising.

The most important consideration in the immediate postoperative period is to remind the patient that the appearance of the treated area will slowly improve over the next several months. The ultimate clinical effect will not be visible at the

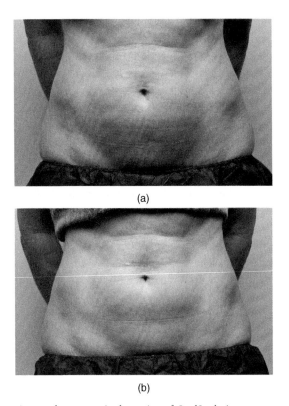

(a)

(b)

Figure 7.12 This patient underwent a single session of CoolSculpting treatment (two applications during the session) to treat the abdomen. Before (a) and 4 months after (b) the treatment, the patient has achieved a significant reduction in the appearance of the excess fat of the abdomen, "the muffin top." (Source: Dr. Flor Mayoral, Coral Gables, FL. Reproduced with permission of Flor Mayoral.)

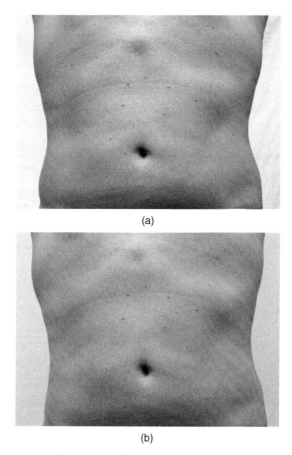

(a)

(b)

Figure 7.13 This patient underwent a single session of CoolSculpting treatment (two applications, one to each flank, during the session) to treat the bilateral "love handles." Before (a) and 6 months after (b) the treatment, the patient has achieved a significant reduction in the appearance of the excess fat of the bilateral flanks, "the love handles." (Source: Dr. Jeffrey Riopelle, San Ramon, CA. Reproduced with permission of Jeffrey Riopelle.)

time of treatment. It is important to schedule a follow-up visit in 2–4 months to evaluate the full effect of the treatment as well as to determine if further treatments may be beneficial (Figures 7.12 and 7.13). Multiple treatments have been shown in clinical studies to further enhance the clinical effects of the procedure.

Summary

Cryolipolysis is a novel, safe, and noninvasive method to reduce the thickness and appearance of subcutaneous fat through controlled cold exposure. Multiple animal studies and human clinical studies have demonstrated the significant visible contour change that occurs following a single cryolipolysis treatment. The treatment is safe, easy, and well-tolerated with no significant adverse events. No cases of scarring, dyspigmentation, or significant alterations in lipid profiles have been reported.

CoolSculpting is a commercially available, FDA cleared device for noninvasive fat reduction utilizing cryolipolysis technology. CoolSculpting is an excellent treatment option for patients seeking noninvasive fat contouring; however, it is not an alternative to liposuction for large volume fat removal. The ideal candidate is a patient with discrete, localized fat bulges. Multiple clinical studies have documented the efficacy of CoolSculpting in the treatment of flank (love handles), back (back fat pads), and abdominal fat (muffin top). Ongoing clinical studies will continue to define the role and efficacy of this procedure for the treatment of unwanted fat in additional areas. As patients continue to desire fat removal and body sculpting, cryolipolysis appears to be a novel method to achieve these goals through a safe, effective, and noninvasive treatment.

References

1 *American Society for Aesthetic Plastic Surgery 2009 Annual Statistics*. Available at: http://www .cosmeticplasticsurgerystatistics.com/statistics.html#2009-HIGHLIGHTS [accessed on 23 June 2011].

2 Rotman, H. (1966) Cold panniculitis in children. *Archives of Dermatology*, **94**, 720–721.

3 Duncan, W.C., Freeman, R.G. & Heaton, C.L. (1966) Cold panniculitis. *Archives of Dermatology*, **94**, 722–724.

4 Beacham, B.E., Cooper, P.H., Buchanan, C.S. *et al* (1980) Equestrian cold panniculitis in women. *Archives of Dermatology*, **116**, 1025–1027.

5 Manstein, D., Laubach, H., Watanabe, K., Farinelli, W., Zurakowski, D. & Anderson, R.R. (2008) Selective cryolysis: a novel method of non-invasive fat removal. *Lasers in Surgery and Medicine*, **40** (**9**), 595–604.

6 Preciado, J. & Allison, J. (2008) The effect of cold exposure on adipocytes: examining a novel method for the noninvasive removal of fat. *Cryobiology*, **57**, 327.

7 Nelson, A.A., Wasserman, D. & Avram, M.M. (2009) Cryolipolysis for reduction of excess adipose tissue. *Seminars in Cutaneous Medicine and Surgery*, **28** (**4**), 244–249.

8 Avram, M.M. & Harry, R.S. (2009) Cryolipolysis for subcutaneous fat layer reduction. *Lasers in Surgery and Medicine*, **41** (**10**), 703–708.

9 Dover, J., Burns, J., Coleman, S. *et al.* (2009) A prospective clinical study of noninvasive cryolipolysis for subcutaneous fat layer reduction – interim report of available subject data. *Presented at the Annual Meeting of the American Society for Laser Medicine and Surgery, April 2009, National Harbor, Maryland.*

10 Kaminer, M., Weiss, R., Newman, J. *et al.* (2009) Visible cosmetic improvement with cryolipolysis: photographic evidence. *Presented at the Annual Meeting of the American Society for Dermatologic Surgery, 2009, Phoenix, AZ.*

11 Rosales-Berber, I.A. & Diliz-Perez, E. (2009) Controlled cooling of subcutaneous fat for body reshaping. *Presented at the 15th World Congress of the International Confederation for Plastic, Reconstructive and Aesthetic Surgery, 2009, New Delhi, India.*

12 Jalian, HR, Avram, MM, Garibyan, L, *et al.* (2014) Paradoxical adipose hyperplasia after cryolipolysis. *JAMA Dermatology,* **150** (**3**), 317–319.

13 Coleman, S.R., Sachdeva, K., Egbert, B.M. *et al.* (2009) Clinical efficacy of noninvasive cryolipolysis and its effects on peripheral nerves. *Aesthetic Plastic Surgery,* **33** (**4**), 482–488.

14 Zelickson, B., Egbert, B.M., Preciado, J. *et al.* (2009) Cryolipolysis for noninvasive fat cell destruction: initial results from a pig model. *Dermatologic Surgery,* **35** (**10**), 1462–1470.

15 Klein, K.B., Zelickson, B., Riopelle, J.G. *et al.* (2009) Non-invasive cryolipolysis for subcutaneous fat reduction does not affect serum lipid levels or liver function tests. *Lasers in Surgery and Medicine,* **41** (**10**), 785–790.

CHAPTER 8

Laser lipolysis and laser-assisted liposuction

Robert A. Weiss[1,2]

[1] Department of Dermatology, University of Maryland School of Medicine, MD, USA
[2] MD Laser Skin Vein Institute, MD, USA

Introduction

Suction-assisted lipectomy or liposuction (SAL) was introduced by the Fischer father and son team of cosmetic surgeons in Italy in 1975 [1, 2]. With their blunt-tipped cannula, multiple incision sites and criss-cross tunneling, the Fischers' techniques paved the way for modifications including Illouz's "wet technique" and Klein's tumescent anesthesia [3]. The transition from general anesthesia to tumescent anesthesia was critical since it reduced side effects such as blood loss, postoperative pain, and bruising at the same time that it increased patient satisfaction [4, 5]. Tumescent anesthesia was developed by a dermatologic surgeon as an alternative to requiring general anesthesia while reducing potential side effects. The tumescent technique thus allowed liposuction to be safely moved from a hospital OR environment to an office setting [6]. Additional methods to facilitate fat removal were developed including internal and external ultrasound-assisted liposuction [7, 8] and power-assisted liposuction (PAL) [9, 10]. Of the three techniques, PAL is more widely used today because of relatively low cost of equipment, easier penetration of fibrous

Fat removal: Invasive and non-invasive body contouring, First Edition. Edited by Mathew M. Avram.

fat, and reduced occurrence of skin burns and seromas that have been reported with ultrasound-assisted technique [11].

   The primary mechanism for fat removal utilizing SAL or PAL is fundamentally a process of mechanical disruption to loosen, dislodge, and suction fat that is surrounded by septae of fibrous tissue. In order to obtain a uniform result, the use of significant shearing force to perforate resistant fibrous tissue and to break up clumps of fat is required. It is a physically demanding procedure for the surgeon as well as risking significant injury along the course of the cannula (without tumescence), and risks of injury to adjacent septa and blood vessels [12]. The resulting trauma can be extensive and in inexperienced hands may lead to nonuniform, uneven retraction and irregular skin tightening, as well as increased bleeding and bruising. With conventional liposuction technique, often multiple punctures are required to gain access to localized stubborn fat deposits, which may further exacerbate the potential unintentional injury. Most agree that minimizing the size of the cannula may decrease the overall trauma to the tissue, but risks of bruising and other side effects cannot be completely eliminated. The smaller the cannula, however, the more tedious the procedure for the surgeon, as more passes are required to free similar volumes of fat.

History of laser lipolysis

Laser lipolysis as an adjunct to liposuction (LAL, laser-assisted liposuction) was conceptually envisioned as a way to minimize potential injury and reduce irregular pockets of remaining fat by melting fat tissue before suctioning removal as well as to reduce the physically demanding requirements for the surgeon. The possible benefits for laser lipolysis include liquefying fat, freeing fat pockets trapped by septae that are impenetrable by a cannula, coagulating small blood vessels, and inducing collagenesis with remodeling with the hope of promoting tissue tightening and retraction [13–16].

   LAL was first described by Dressel [17] in the Lipoplasty Society Newsletter and subsequently investigated by Apfelberg *et al.* [18] in a 51-patient study. In this study, 15 subjects received LAL on one side with the neodymium-doped yttrium–aluminum–garnet (Nd:YAG) laser and 15 received conventional SAL on the contralateral side. The settings for the Nd:YAG laser were 40 W, 0.2-s pulse duration, and a 600 µm fiber inserted into a 4 or 6 mm cannula. This fiber was encased within a cannula and was not in direct contact with the fatty tissue. The study implied decreased ecchymoses, pain, and edema and less effort for the surgeon [18]. While reduced ecchymoses, pain, and edema were demonstrated on the LAL-treated side in comparison with the SAL-treated side, patient results were inconsistent and this particular technique was not cleared for that indication by the U.S. Food and Drug Administration (FDA) [19]. Prado *et al.* [15] examined the efficacy of the 1064 nm Nd:YAG laser in a 25-patient, double-blinded, randomized, controlled, split-body study with LAL performed on one side and SAL on the contralateral side [15]. The only statistically significant difference between the two treatments (LAL vs SAL) was that less pain was observed on the LAL-treated side. Clinical outcomes were comparable for both treatments as evaluated by two independent, blinded-investigators [15]. In another study examining the efficacy of the 1064 nm laser for the treatment of small, discrete areas (focal areas of fat <100 cm^3), LAL treatment was associated with high patient satisfaction, quick recovery times, dermal tightening, and minimal side effects lasting for 1–2 weeks [20]. This study by Kim and Geronemus used magnetic resonance imaging (MRI) to evaluate the volume of fat reduction after laser lipolysis. In addition to the 17% fat volume reduction documented by MRI, patients noted a 37% improvement in only 3 months, quick recovery times, and good skin retraction.

The 2006 study by Goldman [21] also used the 1064 nm laser to reduce submental fat in 82 patients, reporting significant cosmetic improvement with acceptable skin contraction [21]. While no side effects directly related to laser use were reported, the authors did report two cases of asymmetry. A subsequent retrospective study by Goldman in which 1734 patients' treatments were followed including 313 men and 1421 women showed more favorable results [22]. These patients demonstrated less blood loss and bruising, better efficacy for reducing fat in more fibrous regions, and improved comfort postoperatively.

The first laser to be cleared by the FDA for laser lipolysis was a 6 W Nd:YAG laser (Smartlipo™ Cynosure, Westford, MA). Following this clearance for laser fat melting, but not for the term "laser liposuction," many devices and wavelengths were introduced into the medical device arena (Table 8.1). Heavy marketing as well as many influential positive patient and media-related experiences reported online propelled the interest in laser lipolysis procedures.

Table 8.1 Devices for Laser Lipolysis.

Brand Name: Company	Source of laser	Wavelength (nm)	Target	Pulsed (ms) versus continuous
CoolLipo: CoolTouch	Nd:Yag	1320	Water	P
SlimLipo: Palomar	Diode	924/975	Fat – 924 nm Water – 975 nm	C
SmartLipo: Cynosure	Nd:Yag	1064	Water	P
SmartLipo MPX: Cynosure	Nd:Yag	1064/1320	Water	P
SmartLipo Triplex: Cynosure	Nd:Yag	1064/1320/1440	Water	P
ProLipo: Sciton	Nd:Yag	1064/1319	Water	P
LipoLite: Syneron	Nd:Yag	1064	Water	P
Lipotherme: Osyris	Diode	980	Water	C
SmoothLipo: Eleme	Diode	920	Water	C

For the practitioner, a dizzying array of laser wavelengths have all been touted to lead to fat melting and improvement of SAL. In 2007, Mordon *et al.* [23] reported a theoretical model of laser lipolysis combining the use of a 980 nm diode device with a 1064 nm Nd:YAG device. Mordon reported that an internal temperature range of 48–50 °C was required to induce skin tightening. This agreed with the previous report that temperatures of about 45 °C are required for collagen remodeling with energy delivered at the skin surface [24]. This study also suggested that heat, rather than a particular wavelength, led to lipolysis and skin tightening. We have found that wavelengths primarily absorbed by water, while assisting heating the dermis for the goal of skin tightening or retraction are not the optimal wavelengths for laser lipolysis or fat melting. Selectivity for fat is essential when choosing a wavelength for laser lipolysis. While studies have demonstrated that LAL offers increased efficacy for skin retraction and shrinkage through coagulation of the collagen [25], the potential benefits that laser lipolysis may add to liposuction are presently still actively being debated. Much of the confusion surrounding laser lipolysis arises from the promotion of so many wavelengths with more marketing behind them than any science.

Wavelength and pulse duration

Multiple wavelengths, including 924, 968, 980, 1064, 1319, 1320, 1344, and 1440 nm, have all been reported to promote laser lipolysis or fat melting. Table 8.1 lists devices and wavelengths available and their primary target. The best approach for deciding as to which wavelength to utilize is to analyze which wavelengths actually target fat selectively. If fat liquefaction by selective heating is the desired endpoint, then one must analyze and search for wavelengths that are preferentially absorbed by fat compared to water. The objective is to design a device with a lipid-selective laser wavelength rather than a water-selective wavelength. Such a device would allow for controlled, thermal disruption of adipocytes with the least potential injury for the dermis. A water-selective wavelength, however, makes the most sense for the objective of heating of water surrounding connective tissue (collagen) for skin retraction and tightening. Therefore tightening can be maximized with a collagen/water-selective laser wavelength blended in with the lipid-selective laser wavelength. Figure 8.1 shows analysis of fat versus water absorption by use of photospectometry through human fat samples.

A clear selective absorption by fat compared to water is seen in the 924 nm range with peak absorption by water at 980 nm. Of all the wavelengths currently employed for laser lipolysis, 924 nm is currently the only one that is selectively absorbed by fat. This wavelength range for selective fat absorption has been reported by Anderson [26] and confirmed by our clinical experience. The

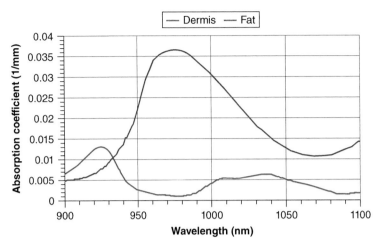

Figure 8.1 Absorption spectrum for fat versus water. Analysis of human fat from abdominoplasty skin. Selective advantage for fat (red line) over water in the 920–925 nm range is observed.

consequences are true enhancement for fat melting with facilitated removal by liposuction. It also implies that, for the best effects for overlying skin contraction, tightening, and stimulation of new collagen, elastin and ground substance heating of the dermis with a water-selective wavelength may be optimal. We have found certain limitations of water targeting wavelengths discussed in side effects below.

Photoacoustic, photomechanical, and photothermal effects are additional theorized mechanisms of action in laser lipolysis. Some have touted photoacoustic effects with microsecond or millisecond pulsing, but newer concepts are based on heating and not on pulse duration [14, 27, 28]. Khoury *et al.* [29] proposed that photoacoustic ablation lends to thermal damage, although photoacoustic damage is difficult to evaluate histologically. It is commonly believed that photoacoustic effects have very little relevance and that straightforward heating of fat is the primary mechanism. To obtain optimal heating, a smooth, continuous power delivery of laser energy is theoretically most effective. Continuous power is predictably safer than energy delivery with high peak-power pulses. Smooth delivery avoids excessively high temperatures, particularly near the output fiber tip. The authors primarily use a dual wavelength system that independently targets lipid and water-based tissues (SlimLipo™, Palomar Medical Technologies, Inc., Burlington, MA), which is cleared by the FDA for the indication of laser-assisted lipolysis. The wavelengths 924 and 975 nm were chosen based on a clear peak in the adipose tissue absorption spectrum at 924 nm and a peak in the water absorption spectrum at 975 nm, respectively [26, 30]. In principle, absorption by the lipids of laser light at this 924 nm wavelength is of the appropriate strength to provide efficient penetration into the adipose tissue yet sufficient heating for the release of intracellular lipids while coagulating rather than tearing the nearby fibrous network needed for tissue tightening. Theoretically, the 975 nm dermal- and hydrated adipose tissue-selective wavelength enables direct targeting of collagen within these structures to provide tissue retraction benefits. Delivery of both these wavelengths of laser light in a continuous wave (CW) power mode potentially results in a safer, more efficacious procedure with potentially superior cosmetic outcomes. Observed treatment benefits of this specifically designed LAL system includes ease of use and enhanced control of laser treatment administration with greater ease and control of subsequent aspiration in comparison to SAL. Laser heating modifies the aspirate viscosity and texture enabling the use of a smaller cannula, which further reduces trauma to the tissue and operator fatigue. These added benefits are significant when compared to our previous experiences with standard SAL and with nonlipid-selective LAL devices and gets closer to our ideal of how laser lipolysis can enhance liposuction (Table 8.2). An experiment in which bovine fat was heated by different wavelengths demonstrate larger area of fat melting with 924 nm as opposed to indirect heating of fat by boiling water for 1320 and 1064 nm (Figure 8.2).

In our initial experience with the 924 nm wavelength, we observed good to excellent improvement across all subjects by 3 months posttreatment in all four categories evaluated [31]. Facility of tip advancement was rated as "extremely easy" or "easy" in 83% of rated treatments. "Good" to "excellent" skin textural improvement was observed in 83% of rated subjects. Additional benefits included reduced operator fatigue and uniformity of treatment. Patients tolerated the procedure well with minimal and transient side effects. Immediate side effects of erythema, bruising, and edema were graded as mild or trace. No long-term side effects were observed. Seventy-eight percent of all subjects were extremely satisfied with the procedure and 89% would perform the procedure again. Eighty-nine percent of subjects felt that their appearance of unwanted

Table 8.2 Ideal properties of laser lipolysis for enhanced liposuction.

- Liquefy fat to facilitate removal
- Overlying skin contraction
  - Effect on septae – cellulite
- Fat volume reduction (small areas) without suction
- Reduced blood loss intraoperatively
- Reduced side effects
  - Bruising
  - Postoperative pain
- Faster recovery time
  - Faster drainage of tumescent through laser channels
- Faster results.

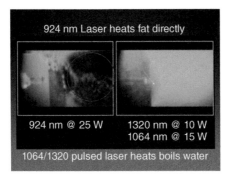

Figure 8.2 An experiment in which bovine fat was heated by two different devices that deliver different wavelengths. At this single frame from a video, there is a larger area of fat melting with 924 nm (circle) as opposed to indirect heating of fat by boiling water by combination of 1320 and 1064 nm (white arrow showing sliver of liquid fat).

fat was significantly improved with smoother and tighter skin (72%), and 94% would recommend the treatment to family and friends.

Indications and patient selection

The primary indication for laser lipolysis with liposuction is body contouring through the liquefaction of localized deposits as well as skin tightening via neo-collagenesis. Laser lipolysis is indicated for many locations with excess adipose tissue and some skin laxity. These include the back hips (muffin-top) submental area, upper extensor arms, abdomen, inner thighs, outer thighs, knees, calves, and ankles. Beyond the standard liposuction candidate/patient, laser lipolysis may play a unique role in certain locations, conditions, or scenarios. For example, fibrous areas, such as the male breast, hips, and back, may be particularly suited for LAL. Our use of 924 nm LAL has enabled treatment of small areas of localized fat in anatomical areas, which have been difficult to treat with SAL. In particular, we were able to achieve fat reduction and skin tightening within a small area of the submentum (Figure 8.3) as well as more precise body contouring and sculpting of upper abdominal regions and of the back containing significant fibrous tissue (Figure 8.3).

The smaller cannula size used for lipolysis may facilitate fat melting in fibrous locations without the additional trauma experienced with larger sized cannulas. Laser lipolysis is also suitable for corrective procedures in which small areas of adiposity may not have been completely removed via previous SAL or other body contouring procedures. Laser disruption has also been reported to facilitate removal of larger lipomas from smaller incisions as well [32].

The advantage of LAL, in our experience, has been that most patients are able to return to normal daily activities within 24–72 h as opposed to 4–7 days with

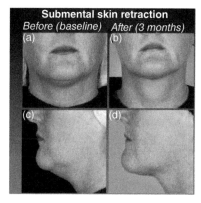

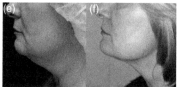

Figure 8.3 Curved surfaces and fibrous areas are particularly suited for laser lipolysis. Submental treatment. Anterior view (a) before and (b) after 6 weeks. Left lateral view (c) before and (d) after 6 weeks. Dramatic tightening/retraction of skin is observed. Clinical results of 924 nm (SlimLipo, Palomar Medical Technologies, Inc. Burlington, MA). (e,f) Similar results are seen with 1320 nm (CoolTouch™, New Star Lasers, Roseville, CA) before and after 6 weeks.

conventional SAL. Laser lipolysis may also diminish postoperative pain, bruising, and edema [33]. Coagulation of blood and lymphatic vessels may explain these advantages. Also previously reported by others, less trauma is required to remove fat due to the liquification of adipose tissue as well as small cannula size [34].

In our experience with several hundred patients, recovery from SAL alone requires 48–72 h of tumescent drainage while after LAL with 924 nm laser, the time is reduced to 12–24 h. The immediate side effects were generally mild or trace in nature and resolved by 2 weeks posttreatment. Similarly, posttreatment pain and discomfort were minimal. In contrast, SAL has historically been associated with significant blood loss, ecchymoses, edema, postoperative pain, and longer recovery time. Likely contributors to these differences between the LAL SAL procedures are the ability to use fewer and smaller incisions and the considerable reduction in tissue trauma arising from use of smaller cannula for aspiration.

These clinical findings demonstrated that the 924/975 nm diode laser system provides safe and efficacious body shaping, fat reduction, and enhanced skin tightening [31]. Ease of movement through the tissue of both the laser system treatment tip and the aspiration cannula resulted in reduced fatigue for the treating physician. Patient benefits included high patient satisfaction, significant reductions in fat, and smoother and tighter skin with minimal downtime.

Laser lipolysis procedure

The basic procedure is the same as tumescent liposuction with tumescent anesthesia injected into the treatment area. This procedure is detailed elsewhere with a detailed discussion of the proper volumes and concentrations of lidocaine [35]. After 30 min of allowing disbursal of tumescence, the laser fiber is inserted into the fat and a fanning motion in the plane of fat layer is performed in order to melt and soften fat. Some prefer to use the laser (especially water targeting) as the last step to heat up skin after the suction is performed. We typically employ seven to nine strokes at 1 cm/s before moving on the next spoke of the fan (Figure 8.4). This is based on some experiments performed at Palomar (data on file) in terms of optimal number of stokes with the 924 nm wavelength.

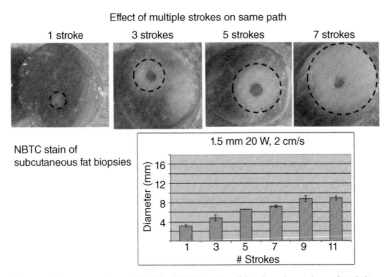

Figure 8.4 Nitroblue tetrazolium chloride (NBTC) stain of fat that shows loss of viability with loss of stain. Every enlarging fat thermal injury as the number of strokes with the laser fiber is increased. This levels off after 9–10 strokes.

Subsequently, suction of "melted" or liberated fat is performed. The aspirate should have an orange color rather than yellow color and contain very little to no chunks of fat. It is important to note that this aspirate cannot be used to inject into other area as there are no living fat cells due to heat destruction (Figure 8.5).

Liquification enhances the ease of removal with 2–3 mm diameter cannulas, and with the submental area as small as 1 mm may be used. Incisions are

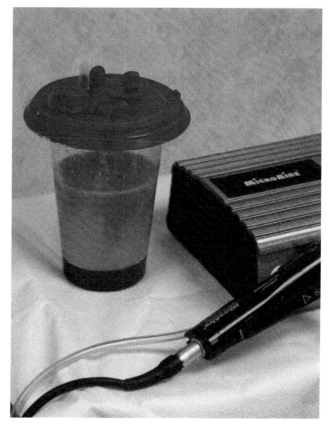

Figure 8.5 Aspirate is homogenized with no chunks of yellow fat but is an orange color and completely liquid after treatment with the 924 nm wavelength. This aspirate cannot be used for lipotransfer as it is acellular. The fat has been removed using a power-assisted liposuction system.

made no more than the size of the cannula to enhance the cosmetic result and speed up healing time. A cycle of laser fat melting liquification and subsequent suction of melted fat is repeated for a second cycle or until tactile sensation or pinching yields significant fat reduction. The fat consistency is monitored with the nondominant hand and after laser heating often feels putty-like with terms such as soft and pliable also used to describe the change in texture. In the process of moving the laser fiber back and forth, we have discovered the creation of a space or plane or "tunnel" for easy removal of tumescent anesthesia. These are visualized in Figure 8.3 after five strokes with the laser fiber. The surgeon and assistants should be able to message the tumescence solution back out at the conclusion of the procedure to facilitate recovery.

Total energies utilized for the laser range from 5000 to 60,000 J/cm^2. Size of the treatment location, the total amount of fat, the number of strokes, distance of cannula placement from the skin and depth within the fat layer, number of repeated cycles passes, and individual surgical techniques prevent recommending an absolute number of kilojoules for each region. Reynaud [36] has published guidelines using a 980 nm diode laser. His average total for each area are 24,600 J for the abdomen, 21,900 J for the back, 14,600 J for the hip, 13,100 J for the buttock, 8100 J for the knee, and 10,400 J for the inner thigh. The cumulative total for the submandibular region seems to be bit high in our experience, since we typically use about 50% of the total of 11,700 J reported.

Complications

The primary complication is from the placement of heat into the fat layer, then greatly reducing the fat layer by liposuction and thereby causing the laser fiber to be closer to the skin on subsequent passes. During later passes after suction has been performed is the time when the most risk of overheating the skin and causing a burn is the highest. Some wavelengths penetrate more deeply and can be more hazardous, such as 1064 nm. The wrong angle of attack through fat may allow the fiber to poke a hole through the skin. As many surgeons perform suction aspiration in addition to laser lipolysis, the procedural time may be significantly increased depending on what device and wavelengths are utilized.

Overall, the disadvantages of laser lipolysis include many of the same side effects following SAL, such as bruising and tenderness. However, significant additional complications are possible including skin injury due to wavelength, pulse duration, tip design, and fiber breakage under the skin of small glass fibers. The use of thicker, flexible fibers with a larger diameter renders the risk of broken fibers negligible. We prefer a fiber of at least 1.5 mm in diameter to deliver the laser energy. In 2008, Katz [37] reported complications associated with laser-assisted lipolysis in 537 cases between January 2006 and November 2007. There were no systemic adverse events. One patient developed a localized infection treated with oral antibiotics and four patients developed burns. The reported side effect profile from our clinic is shown in Table 8.3 [31].

An additional concern is the theoretical possibility of nerve injury. An early histologic study using 1064 nm showed histologically intact nerve fibers within heated and fragmented adipose tissue [22]. Nerve fiber or sensor injury has not been reported in the literature for laser lipolysis with no numbness or paresthesias reported over 2000 cases [34]. Another issue of concern for many patients and for the FDA with the focused ultrasound devices for fat dissolution from the surface is the possibility of increased serum lipids as a result of lipolyzed adipose tissue. No significant change in triglycerides and lipid profiles among patients treated with laser lipolysis or any other liposuction procedure has been reported either short- or long-term [22, 38]. In fact, it appears that serum lipids may decrease several months after liposuction [39, 40].

Table 8.3 Prevalence of immediate and long-term side effects.

Side effects	Immediate	3 months
Skin burns	0	0
Hyperpigmentation	0	0
Erythema	16 (84%)	0
Bruising	14 (74%)	0
Edema	15 (76%)	0
Burn	1 (5%)	0
Asymmetry	1 (5%)	0
Anesthesia – partial	4 (21%)	0
Pain	6 (32%)	0
Allergic reaction to compression garment	1 (5%)	0

Several measures have been reported to enhance the safety of laser lipolysis and specifically reduce thermal injury. An infrared thermometer is sometimes employed to monitor temperature during laser administration to avoid reaching surface temperatures exceeding 45 °C. Above this temperature at the skin surface may result in epidermal and dermal injury as previously reported [24]. A combination of palpation and monitoring skin temperature with the nondominant hand are used during LAL to minimize complications. During lasing, the tissue is continually palpated until it becomes softer putty-like and more supple than at the start of the procedure. Many clinicians also pinch the skin to elevate it allowing better access to subcutaneous fat as shown in Figure 8.6.

Pinching the skin is also used to evaluate the treatment area after laser softening and melting of fat to ensure a smooth and even removal of fatty tissue. For the final pass, no pinching is applied in order to treat more superficially. More specifically, the skin is often stretched with the pass of the laser fiber just below the skin to allow more surface area to be heated safely.

Skin effects

Cumulative data including clinical observation, histological evidence, MRI measurements, and tattoo grid reductions in surface area have led to the conclusion by most of them, who perform laser lipolysis on a regular basis that laser lipolysis has been proven to have an additive effect to liposuction [34]. The most thorough evaluation for skin tightening was a study of the 1064/1320 nm laser in which five patients had placement of 4 cm × 4 cm grid of tattoos for measurement of skin tightening by calculation of surface area. This was accompanied by histology with H&E staining as well as electron microscopy. Biopsies were performed before and 3 days and 1 month after the procedure within at the treated

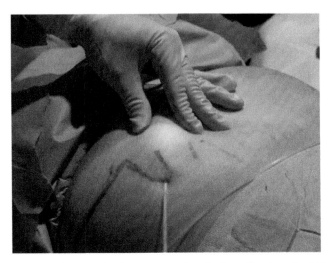

Figure 8.6 Pinching or elevating the skin to insure that the laser fiber is well within fat and cannot poke through the skin. The laser pattern emitted from the tip in a radial manner is seen with this infrared sensing camera. This is the pattern of the 924 nm × 1.5 mm conical fiber tip design.

areas [41]. Electron microscopy demonstrated new collagen formation compared to baseline. No adverse events were reported in this study, while results showed reduction in localized fat deposits as well as an 18% decrease in surface area by tattoo grid measurements indicating a significant skin tightening effect. We have seen until 25% reduction in skin surface area within preexisting periumbilical tattoos (Figure 8.7). In our experience, skin tightening continues to improve for until 6 months after LAL.

Another recent study examined the effects of 1064/1320 nm for skin tightening, with additional of laser on one side of the abdomen compared to liposuction alone on the contralateral side [42]. Ten subjects were included in this study to evaluate skin shrinkage through photographic imaging and measurement of temporary ink markings. Skin tightening was also measured with an elasticity device. Data points included baseline, 1 month, and 3 months posttreatment. The results demonstrated more skin shrinkage on the laser-treated side than on the suction side both at the 1- and 3-month evaluations, although both sides demonstrated improvement. In addition to skin tightening and retraction, our clinical experience is that the addition of laser lipolysis results in smoother more even texture especially over curved surfaces such as flanks with less effort (Figure 8.8). This potentially speeds up the procedure and provides a lot less strain on the physician with less risks of streaking from cannula strokes.

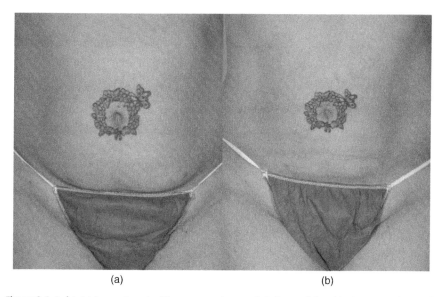

(a)   (b)

Figure 8.7 (a,b) At 3 months, significant retraction or shrinkage of the skin (24%) is observed by measuring the dimensions of a preexisting periumbilical tattoo. Approximately 800 cm^3 of aspirate was removed from this abdomen. A total energy of 60 kJ was delivered using a combination of 924/975 nm.

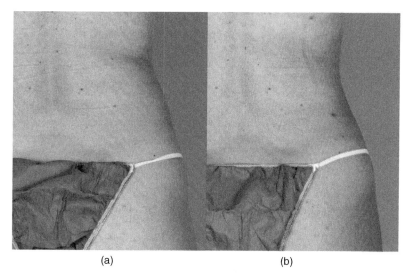

(a)   (b)

Figure 8.8 Laser lipolysis results in smoother more even texture especially over curved surfaces such as flanks with less effort. (a) Before and (b) after 6 weeks showing smooth results with curved and fibrous areas. Laser lipolysis with liposuction eliminated the "muffin-top" seen above the waistline with tight jeans. This patient is in her early 1940s. A total of 20 kJ per flank was delivered using a combination of 924/975 nm.

Summary

At this time, the beneficial effects of laser lipolysis as an adjunct to liposuction remains controversial with many surgeons having had a poor experience with longer procedure time and learning curve of new equipment. We have observed, however, in hundreds of patients, several advantages of using laser for fat melting including facilitated extraction by suction through smaller cannulas. In experienced hands, laser lipolysis provides safe and efficacious body shaping, fat reduction, and enhanced skin tightening or retraction. Choice of wavelength is critical and understanding the interaction of the wavelength with fat is important. Once fat melting and softening is achieved with laser, the ease of movement through the tissue of both the laser system treatment tip and the aspiration cannula results in reduced fatigue for the treating physician. Procedure time may be reduced especially in difficult areas. Fibrous areas, such as the male breast, or curved areas such as female hips and back, may be particularly suited for laser lipolysis. Previous liposuction patients with increased fibrous tissue are good candidates as well. Patient benefits include reduction of downtime high accompanied by high patient satisfaction, significant reductions in fat, and smoother and tighter skin.

References

1 Fischer, G. (1990) Liposculpture: the "correct" history of liposuction. Part I. *The Journal of Dermatologic Surgery and Oncology*, **16**, 1087–1089.

2 Klein, J.A. (1988) Anesthesia for liposuction in dermatologic surgery. *The Journal of Dermatologic Surgery and Oncology*, **14**, 1124–1132.

3 Illouz, Y.G. (1984) Illouz's technique of body contouring by lipolysis. *Clinics in Plastic Surgery*, **11**, 409–417.

4 Klein, J.A. (1990) Tumescent technique for regional anesthesia permits lidocaine doses of 35 mg/kg for liposuction. *The Journal of Dermatologic Surgery and Oncology*, **16**, 248–263.

5 Klein, J.A. (1993) Tumescent technique for local anesthesia improves safety in large-volume liposuction. *Plastic and Reconstructive Surgery*, **92**, 1085–1098; discussion 1099–1100.

6 Coleman, W.P. 3rd. (1990) The history of liposculpture. *The Journal of Dermatologic Surgery and Oncology*, **16**, 1086.

7 Zocchi, M.L. (1996) Ultrasonic assisted lipoplasty. Technical refinements and clinical evaluations. *Clinics in Plastic Surgery*, **23**, 575–598.

8 Silberg, B.N. (1998) The use of external ultrasound assist with liposuction. *Aesthetic Surgery Journal/The American Society for Aesthetic Plastic Surgery*, **18**, 284–285.

9 Rebelo, A. (2006) Power-assisted liposuction. *Clinics In Plastic Surgery*, **33**, 91–105 vii.

10 Fodor, P.B. (2005) Power-assisted lipoplasty versus traditional suction-assisted lipoplasty: comparative evaluation and analysis of output. *Aesthetic Plastic Surgery*, **29**, 127.

11 Coleman, W.P. 3rd. (2000) Powered liposuction. *Dermatologic Surgery*, **26**, 315–318.

12 Blondeel, P.N., Derks, D., Roche, N., Van Landuyt, K.H. & Monstrey, S.J. (2003) The effect of ultrasound-assisted liposuction and conventional liposuction on the perforator vessels in the lower abdominal wall. *British Journal of Plastic Surgery*, **56**, 266–271.

13 Goldman, A. & Gotkin, R.H. (2009) Laser-assisted liposuction. *Clinics in Plastic Surgery*, **36**, 241–253 vii; discussion 255–260.

14 Goldman, A., Wollina, U. & de Mundstock, E.C. (2011) Evaluation of tissue tightening by the subdermal Nd: YAG laser-assisted liposuction versus liposuction alone. *Journal of Cutaneous and Aesthetic Surgery*, **4**, 122–128.

15 Prado, A., Andrades, P., Danilla, S., Leniz, P., Castillo, P. & Gaete, F. (2006) A prospective, randomized, double-blind, controlled clinical trial comparing laser-assisted lipoplasty with suction-assisted lipoplasty. *Plastic and Reconstructive Surgery*, **118**, 1032–1045.

16 Sasaki, G.H. & Tevez, A. (2009) Laser-assisted liposuction for facial and body contouring and tissue tightening: a 2-year experience with 75 consecutive patients. *Seminars in Cutaneous Medicine and Surgery*, **28**, 226–235.

17 Dressel, T. (1990) Laser lipoplasty: a preliminary report. *Lipoplasty Society Newsletter*, **7**, 17.

18 Apfelberg, D.B., Rosenthal, S., Hunstad, J.P., Achauer, B. & Fodor, P.B. (1994) Progress report on multicenter study of laser-assisted liposuction. *Aesthetic Plastic Surgery*, **18**, 259–264.

19 Apfelberg, D.B. (1996) Results of multicenter study of laser-assisted liposuction. *Clinics in Plastic Surgery*, **23**, 713–719.

20 Kim, K.H. & Geronemus, R.G. (2006) Laser lipolysis using a novel 1,064 nm Nd:YAG Laser. *Dermatologic Surgery: Official Publication for American Society for Dermatologic Surgery [et al]*, **32**, 241–248 discussion 247.

21 Goldman, A. (2006) Submental Nd:Yag laser-assisted liposuction. *Lasers in Surgery and Medicine*, **38**, 181–184.

22 Goldman, A., Schavelzon, D. & Blugerman, G. (2002) Laser lipolysis: liposuction with Nd:YAG laser. *Revista da Sociedade Brasileira de Laser Medicine*, **2**, 15–17.

23 Mordon, S.R., Wassmer, B., Reynaud, J.P. & Zemmouri, J. (2008) Mathematical modeling of laser lipolysis. *Biomedical Engineering Online*, **7**, 10.

24 Fatemi, A., Weiss, M.A. & Weiss, R.A. (2002) Short-term histologic effects of nonablative resurfacing: results with a dynamically cooled millisecond-domain 1320 nm Nd:YAG laser. *Dermatologic Surgery: Official Publication for American Society for Dermatologic Surgery [et al]*, **28**, 172–176.

25 Badin, A.Z., Moraes, L.M., Gondek, L., Chiaratti, M.G. & Canta, L. (2002) Laser lipolysis: flaccidity under control. *Aesthetic Plastic Surgery*, **26**, 335–339.

26 Anderson, R.R., Farinelli, W., Laubach, H. *et al.* (2006) Selective photothermolysis of lipid-rich tissues: a free electron laser study. *Lasers in Surgery and Medicine*, **38**, 913–919.

27 Sadick, N.S., Diktaban, T. & Smoller, B.R. (2010) New clinical outcomes utilizing a 1064-nm Nd:YAG laser for lipolysis of the torso oblique region. *Journal of Cosmetic and Laser Therapy: Official Publication of the European Society for Laser Dermatology*, **12**, 170–175.

28 Sasaki, G.H. (2010) Quantification of human abdominal tissue tightening and contraction after component treatments with 1064-nm/1320-nm laser-assisted lipolysis: clinical implications. *Aesthetic Surgery Journal/The American Society for Aesthetic Plastic Surgery*, **30**, 239–245.

29 Khoury, J.G., Saluja, R., Keel, D., Detwiler, S. & Goldman, M.P. (2008) Histologic evaluation of interstitial lipolysis comparing a 1064, 1320 and 2100 nm laser in an ex vivo model. *Lasers in Surgery and Medicine*, **40**, 402–406.

30 O'Dey, D., Prescher, A., Poprawe, R., Gaus, S., Stanzel, S. & Pallua, N. (2008) Ablative targeting of fatty-tissue using a high-powered diode laser. *Lasers in Surgery and Medicine*, **40**, 100–105.

31 Weiss, R.A. & Beasley, K. (2009) Laser-assisted liposuction using a novel blend of lipid- and water-selective wavelengths. *Lasers in Surgery and Medicine*, **41**, 760–766.

32 Stebbins, W.G., Hanke, C.W. & Petersen, J. (2011) Novel method of minimally invasive removal of large lipoma after laser lipolysis with 980 nm diode laser. *Dermatologic Therapy*, **24**, 125–130.

33 Palm, M.D. & Goldman, M.P. (2009) Laser lipolysis: current practices. *Seminars in Cutaneous Medicine and Surgery*, **28**, 212–219.

34 McBean, J.C. & Katz, B.E. (2011) Laser lipolysis: an update. *The Journal of Clinical and Aesthetic Dermatology*, **4**, 25–34.

35 Klein, J.A. (1999) Anesthetic formulation of tumescent solutions. *Dermatologic Clinics*, **17**, 751–759 v–vi.

36 Reynaud, J.P., Skibinski, M., Wassmer, B., Rochon, P. & Mordon, S. (2009) Lipolysis using a 980-nm diode laser: a retrospective analysis of 534 procedures. *Aesthetic Plastic Surgery*, **33**, 28–36.

37 Katz, B. & McBean, J. (2008) Laser-assisted lipolysis: a report on complications. *Journal of Cosmetic and Laser Therapy: Official Publication of the European Society for Laser Dermatology*, **10**, 231–233.

38 Scuderi, N., Paolini, G., Grippaudo, F.R. & Tenna, S. (2000) Comparative evaluation of traditional, ultrasonic, and pneumatic assisted lipoplasty: analysis of local and systemic effects, efficacy, and costs of these methods. *Aesthetic Plastic Surgery*, **24**, 395–400.

39 Giese, S.Y., Bulan, E.J., Commons, G.W., Spear, S.L. & Yanovski, J.A. (2001) Improvements in cardiovascular risk profile with large-volume liposuction: a pilot study. *Plastic and Reconstructive Surgery*, **108**, 510–519; discussion 520–511.

40 Baxter, R.A. (1997) Serum lipid changes following large-volume suction lipectomy. *Aesthetic Surgery Journal/The American Society for Aesthetic Plastic Surgery*, **17**, 213–215.

41 McBean, J.C. & Katz, B.E. (2009) A pilot study of the efficacy of a 1,064 and 1,320 nm sequentially firing Nd:YAG laser device for lipolysis and skin tightening. *Lasers in Surgery and Medicine*, **41**, 779–784.

42 DiBernardo, B.E. & Reyes, J. (2009) Evaluation of skin tightening after laser-assisted liposuction. *Aesthetic Surgery Journal/The American Society for Aesthetic Plastic Surgery*, **29**, 400–407.

CHAPTER 9

Soft tissue augmentation for facial lipoatrophy and volumization

Nazanin Saedi[1] and Kenneth Arndt[2,3,4,5]

[1] Laser Surgery and Cosmetic Dermatology, Thomas Jefferson University, PA, USA

[2] SkinCare Physicians, MA, USA

[3] Harvard Medical School, MA, USA

[4] Brown University, RI, USA

[5] The Geisel School of Medicine at Dartmouth, NH, USA

Introduction

Over the past decade, dermal fillers have provided a safe and effective means for aesthetic soft tissue augmentation and have experienced a dramatic increase in popularity. Fillers are used to soften superficial wrinkles, minimize deep folds, and restore volume on the face. The filler revolution started with collagen, and, subsequently extended to hyaluronic acid (HA) fillers and has paved the way for the development of biostimulatory materials [1]. The appropriate selection of an agent depends on the size, depth, and location of the volume deficiency.

Hyaluronic acid derivatives

The HA derivatives continue to be the most widely used fillers for soft tissue augmentation. HA is an acid mucopolysaccharide that resides in the cutaneous dermal ground substance and fills the extracellular spaces between collagen fibers. It is a ubiquitous component of the connective tissue matrix in the dermis,

Fat removal: Invasive and non-invasive body contouring, First Edition. Edited by Mathew M. Avram.
© 2015 John Wiley & Sons, Ltd. Published 2015 by John Wiley & Sons, Ltd.

and its main biologic function is to create volume and lubricate extracellular structures. HA acts as a scaffold for collagen and elastin to bind. As the skin loses HA with aging, there is decreased movement and elasticity. As HA, consists of repeating polymer chains of the polysaccharide with interval cross-links of agents that bind the polymers together, it used in commercial filler agents.

The hydrophilic nature of HA means that the more concentrated products will tend to imbibe more water, and thus have more tissue swelling following injection. After an equilibrium is reached with the surrounding tissue, more concentrated products will maintain more swelling and fullness in the treated area [2]. Characteristics that make each HA product unique include cross-linking, concentration of the HA, amount of free HA (non-cross-linked), granule size, and G′ prime (lift factor) [3, 4].

The commonly used injectable HAs are produced by streptococcal fermentation (nonanimal stabilized hyaluronic acid, NASHA). In the Restylane® family (Galderma, Switzerland), the following forms are available: Restylane-L® and Perlane-L®. Both the forms contain 0.3% lidocaine to ease the pain of the injection. Each has a concentration of 20 mg/mL of HA, but the difference is the size of the gel particles. Restylane has 100,000 gel particles per milliliter, and is U.S. Food and Drug Administration (FDA) approved for deep wrinkle correction, lip augmentation, nasolabial fold correction, and for glabellar creases. Restylane has been used with success for the treatment of tear trough deformities [5]. Perlane® (8000 gel particles per milliliter) is for deep dermal augmentation and the more profound facial folds. Postinjection swelling, erythema, and bruising are not atypical and may be more prolonged than with other HA fillers. When comparing small particle gels and large particle gels, they both demonstrate similar efficacy, durability, and safety [6]. Perlane has also been shown to be effective for the treatment of HIV lipoatrophy. Gooderham and Solish [7] reported using 5–6 cm^3 in total of the HA in the malar area with intradermal injection. At the 6-month follow-up, sustained longevity was observed. Bugge *et al.* [8] in Norway studied HA for the treatment of facial fat atrophy in HIV-positive patients and used Restylane SubQ, which is a larger particle Restylane product. Twenty-seven patients were treated in each cheek at baseline, 12 months, and then 24 months. The intended level of injection was the deep subcutaneous fat. Patients classified their facial appearance as very much improved or moderately improved, and they reported increased satisfaction with their facial appearance along with higher self-esteem scores.

Juvederm® (Allergan Inc., Irvine, CA) is similar to Restylane in that it is based on nonanimal, cross-linked technology. There are similarly three forms: Juvederm (18 mg/mL of HA), Juvederm Ultra (24 mg/mL of HA) for deeper mid-dermal defects, and Juvederm Ultra Plus (30 mg/mL of HA) for correction of the deepest contour irregularities [2]. The two thicker forms, Juvederm Ultra and Juvederm Ultra Plus, were granted FDA approval in 2007. One formulation of Juvederm, recently FDA approved in the United States, is Juvederm Voluma, which is intended for midface volumizing, where a high lift capacity and larger volumes are required. Voluma is a more viscous product with a robust lift capacity. Voluma, which was approved for use in Europe, Canada, and Australia before approval in the United States, may play an important role in treating lipoatrophy. Raspaldo [9] assessed the effectiveness and safety of Voluma in maintaining increased volume in the malar area for up to 18 months posttreatment. Retrospective record data was analyzed for 102 patients (93 females, 9 males; mean age: 51.27 years), who received Voluma injected into the midface. All patients were assessed at baseline and at 1 month and 6–18 months postinjection. Voluma provided aesthetic improvements according to investigator and patient assessment for up to 18 months posttreatment with an excellent safety profile. Other studies have also documented excellent results with Voluma for age-related and HIV-related mid-facial lipoatrophy [10, 11].

Soft tissue augmentation using available HA derivatives lasts approximately 6–12 months, longer than most of the other temporary fillers [12]. Adverse reactions include ecchymosis, acneiform eruptions, and reactivation of herpes simplex [13, 14]. Injection discomfort, postinjection ache, erythema, and edema are expected sequelae. With most fillers, if the placement is too superficial, a contour irregularity results and the resolution occurs only with time. However, with HA, a "lump" can often be redistributed into the desired location by physician massage. If is the lump persists, the irregularity can be treated with various methods. The material can be expressed by simple incision and drainage. With manual pressure, the clear intact hyaluronan is readily extruded. If the administration has been too deep and the localized bump is not readily accessible to drainage, local injection of small amount of hyaluronidase can reduce its size. When the product is placed too superficially, it causes the formation of a blue-gray cutaneous bead known as the Tyndall effect, which is created because of different wavelengths of light scattering depending on the size of the substance that they encounter. In the skin, longer red wavelengths penetrate deeper into the tissue while the shorter blue wavelengths are scattered and reflected outward [15]. Fortunately, this complication also responds to the intralesional injection of hyaluronidase [16]. All of the HA products may create a Tyndall effect except for Belotero® (Merz, San Mateo, CA).

True hypersensitivity to injectable HA is rare, and occurs in about 1/5000 cases [17]. Infection is quite uncommon as well and can usually be managed with either antibiotics or antivirals depending on the clinical features. Biofilms are hypothesized to cause rare nodular reaction to HA injection.

The complication of greatest concern is cutaneous necrosis, which is most commonly caused by occlusion of vascular structures by inadvertent injection of HA intravascularly or by sidewall compression of vascular structures due to overvolumizing of the surrounding soft tissue. The supratrochlear artery in the glabellar area and the angular artery in the superior nasolabial fold are particularly susceptible. Necrosis leads to retiform purpura, and, if untreated, leads to potential ulceration and scar. The injecting physician should have knowledge of vascular structures in the areas of injection. Further, treatment endpoints such as whitening or purpuric discoloration should be observed carefully.

Calcium hydroxylapatite

Calcium hydroxylapatite (CaHA), Radiesse® (Merz, San Mateo, CA), was initially approved for laryngoplasty (vocal cords) and stress-related bladder sphincter incompetence. It has found a niche in the filler market because its duration is estimated to be up to 1–2 years with some reports that it may last 2–5 years [18]. It is a milky white suspension comprised of two components: (i) an aqueous gel carrier containing glycerin, sodium carboxymethylcellulose, and water and (ii) the matrix particle. Once the carrier dissipates, the matrix, composed of 25–125 µm microspheres of CaHA, provides the augmentation effect. CaHA is a nonallergenic (inert) bioceramic that is identical to the primary mineral constituents found in bone and teeth. The material is deposited deeply at the dermal–subcutaneous junction. This product stimulates neocollagenesis around the injected microspheres, which are eventually degraded over several years. As the CaHA implant is radiopaque, the patient should be informed that it might be visible on dental radiographs. This product was approved in 2006 for the correction of facial wrinkles and folds and also for HIV-associated facial lipoatrophy. Off-label facial uses also include correction of marionette lines and oral commissures, the prejowl sulcus, midface volume loss, dorsal nasal deformities, and chin augmentation.

In order to treat HIV-treated lipoatrophy and more advanced facial lipoatrophy associated with age or lean body mass, a sufficient volume of CaHA needs to be used. In a study on the use of CaHA for HIV facial lipoatrophy, the authors described optimal correction as "very much improved" on the Global Aesthetic Improvement Score (GAIS) and sought to determine the volume necessary to achieve the optimal correction. Thirty patients were treated with CaHA injections into the subdermal and supramuscular planes in the submalar region. The average initial treatment volume was 9.5 mL per patient (both sides) and the total volume per patient after 12 months averaged 16.1 mL. Eighty percent (24) patients achieved the GAIS score of the "very much improved" at 3 months and 60% (18) at 6 months [19]. When lower volumes of CaHA were used, the patients did not see as much improvement, highlighting the importance of using sufficient volume to correct lipoatrophy [20].

Poly-L-lactic acid

Polymerized polylactic acid (PPLA) is a powdered lyophilized suture material, that is, Vicryl® (polyglactin 910). Freeze-dried preparations of polylactic acid are stored at room temperature, and, before injection, each vial must be reconstituted with sterile water. A 26-gauge needle is used to place the product high in the subcutaneous/deep dermal plane without overcorrection. There may be the appearance of some immediate augmentation due to edema, but in order to achieve dermal thickness and prolonged neocollagenesis, the recommended protocol is a series of three to four injections at 3- to 6-week intervals. Persistence of augmentation has varied, but some improvement has been seen to last over 2 years. In 2004, a PPLA, Sculptra® (Valeant Pharmaceuticals, Bridgewater, NJ), was FDA-approved for the correction of shape and contour deficiencies resulting from facial lipoatrophy associated with highly active antiretroviral therapy (HAART) for HIV-infected patients [21]. In 2009, Sculptra was approved by the FDA for use in volumization of the aging face. It was approved for the correction of shallow to deep nasolabial folds, contour deficiencies, and other facial wrinkles and lines.

In 2003, the pilot study on poly-L-lactic acid (PLLA) for HIV facial lipoatrophy was a 96-week, uncontrolled, single-center, open-label study, and 50 HIV-infected patients received antiretroviral therapy with PLLA at 2-week intervals for 6 weeks. No severe treatment-related adverse events were encountered; however, 52% of patients developed palpable but nonvisible and nonbothersome subcutaneous nodules. The patients were evaluated by clinical examination, photographs, and ultrasonography, and results included significant increases in total cutaneous thickness with improved facial aesthetics and improved quality of life.

As more experience with the product was determined by clinical practice, it was found that increasing dilution and placement of the product in deeper planes than the dermis decreased the incidence of subcutaneous papules. A review of the literature by Kates and Fitzgerald [22] showed that the rates of papule formation had fallen to 0–13% using newer protocols for treatment. At present, the recommended dilution of the product with 5 mL or more of sterile water and the addition of lidocaine, 1–2%, to achieve a final dilution of 8–9 mL per vial [23]. Injections should be placed in the superficial subcutaneous or preperiosteal planes. Patients are instructed to massage the injected regions for 5 min, five times a day for 5 days after treatment.

Permanent filler – silicone for HIV lipoatrophy

Silicone, polydimethylsiloxane, consists of repeating units of dimethylsiloxane terminated with trimethylsiloxane. Centistoke (cST) is a measure of viscosity and silicone viscosity is directly related to the chain length of the repeating units. A 1 cST product is equivalent in consistency to water, 350 cST products are oils similar in consistency to mineral oils, and a 1000-cST product is similar in texture to honey. Pure injectable-grade liquid silicone was never approved by the FDA and remains prohibited in the United States. However, injectable intraocular silicone (AdatoSil® 5000 cST) was approved in 1994 for tamponade to treat complicated retinal detachment. Silikon 1000® was approved for intraocular use in 1997. In 2001, the FDA approved a clinical study of SilSkin®, a highly purified 1000-cST oil, for the treatment of nasolabial folds, marionette lines, and mid-malar depressions. In 2003, the FDA also approved SilSkin for investigational treatment of HIV-associated lipoatrophy.

As the placement of the product results in permanent augmentation, there is very little margin for error, and meticulous technique is essential. Many practitioners prefer to use a glass syringe attached to a 27- or 30-gauge needle. The silicone is deposited using a microdroplet serial puncture technique, using 0.005–0.01 mL aliquots placed at 2–5 mm intervals within the dermis without overcorrection. Each treatment should not exceed 0.5 mL of silicone for treating small areas and 2 mL for the treatment of HIV lipoatrophy [24]. The intervals between sessions are usually monthly until the collagen response and cumulative fibroplasia achieve the desired result. As the endpoint of treatment approaches, the volume injected per visit diminishes and the time interval between treatments lengthens.

Common posttreatment events include erythema, edema, and ecchymosis. The incidence of overcorrection with superficial beading, granulomatous reactions, and inflammatory reactions has improved based on use of only FDA-approved product and adherence to the microdroplet technique [25, 26].

Polymethylmethacrylate

Injectable polymethylmethacrylate (PMMA), ArteFill® (Suneva, San Diego, CA), is a suspension of 20% PMMA smooth microspheres in 80% bovine collagen. ArteFill is the product of third-generation PMMA microsphere technology. Previous generations include Arteplast® (used in Germany from 1989 to 1994) and Artecoll® (used worldwide, except in the United States and Japan, from 1994 to 2006). Artefill represents a third-generation product containing few nanoparticles (<20 μm), which were thought to be associated with granulomatous reactions observed with previous generations. ArteFill was approved by the FDA in 2006 for the correction of nasolabial folds.

After PMMA is injected, the collagen vehicle is absorbed within 1–3 months. Afterward, new collagen is deposited by the host to encapsulate and engulf the remaining estimated 6 million PMMA particles in 1 mL of ArteFill. This process contributes to tissue augmentation through fibroplasia. Although the collagen is absorbed, the PMMA is permanent and not reabsorbed. Patients should be evaluated 4–6 weeks after the injection to assess the need for further treatments. Optimal correction usually requires two to three treatments, and touch-up implantations should be at intervals of at least 2 weeks or longer depending on the amount of implant used, the site of placement, and the dynamics of the corrected sites.

Injectable PMMA is contraindicated for use in patients with a positive result to the required ArteFill skin test, patients with severe allergies (as indicated by a history of anaphylaxis or multiple severe allergies), patients with known lidocaine hypersensitivity, patients with a history of allergies to bovine collagen products, and patients with known susceptibility to keloid or hypertrophic scarring. Superficial injections should be avoided in order to prevent permanent skin surface texture or color change. There is a risk of a hypersensitivity reaction and delayed granuloma formation.

The pivotal US clinical trial for ArteFill was a controlled, randomized, prospective study of 251 patients [27]. Patients received either ArteFill or bovine collagen dermal filler (control). Efficacy was rated by blinded observers using a photographic Facial Fold Assessment Scale. The study demonstrated a significant improvement with ArteFill compared with the control group at 6 months in nasolabial folds. A subset of patients was observed at 12 months and all showed persistent wrinkle correction. A subgroup of 69 patients were contacted 4–5 years later for further assessment and were evaluated for delayed adverse events. Five patients reported six late adverse events that occurred from 2 to 5 years after the initial injection. Of these, four were mild cases of lumpiness, and two were severe [28].

Conclusion

The vast array of available filler products, and those that are on the horizon, are only one means to improve tissue loss associated with aging and lipoatrophy. Keeping abreast of advances and perfecting a few techniques will be most advantageous for patients; it is not only what is injected, but also how it is injected, which determines the degree of success. Regardless of the treatment chosen, it is the combination of clinical judgment, realistic expectations, meticulous preparation, and surgical skill that provides optimal results.

References

1 Kontis, T.C. (2013) Contemporary review of injectable facial fillers. *JAMA Facial Plastic Surgery*, 1–7. **15** (**1**): 58–64
2 Gilbert, E., Hui, A. & Waldorf, H.A. (2012) The basic science of dermal fillers: past and present. Part I: background and mechanisms of action. *Journal of Drugs in Dermatology*, **11** (**9**), 1059–1068.

3 Tezel, A. & Fredrickson, G.H. (2008) The science of hyaluronic acid dermal fillers. *Journal of Cosmetic and Laser Therapy*, **10** (**1**), 35–42.

4 Falcone, S.J. & Berg, R.A. (2008) Crosslinked hyaluronic acid dermal fillers: a comparison of rheological properties. *Journal of Biomedical Materials Research. Part A*, **87** (**1**), 264–271.

5 Gold, M.H. (2007) Use of hyaluronic acid fillers for the treatment of the aging face. *Clinical Interventions in Aging*, **2** (**3**), 369–376.

6 Dover, J.S., Rubin, M.G. & Bhatia, A.C. (2009) Review of the efficacy, durability, and safety data of two nonanimal stabilized hyaluronic acid fillers from a prospective, randomized, comparative, multicenter study. *Dermatologic Surgery*, **35**, 322–331.

7 Gooderham, M. & Solish, N. (2005) Use of hyaluronic acid for soft tissue augmentation of HIV-associated facial lipodystrophy. *Dermatologic Surgery*, **31** (**1**), 104–108.

8 Bugge, H., Negaard, A., Skeie, L. & Bergersen, B. (2007) Hyaluronic acid treatment of facial fat atrophy in HIV-positive patients. *HIV Medicine*, **8** (**8**), 475–482.

9 Raspaldo, H. (2008) Volumizing effect of a new hyaluronic acid sub-dermal facial filler: a retrospective analysis based on 102 cases. *Journal of Cosmetic and Laser Therapy*, **10** (**3**), 134–142.

10 Carruthers, J. & Carruthers, A. (2010) Volumizing with a 20 mg/mL smooth, highly cohesive, viscous hyaluronic acid filler and its role in facial rejuvenation therapy. *Dermatologic Surgery*, **36** (**3**), 1886–1892.

11 Jones, D. (2010) A new option for facial volume: volumizing with a 20 mg/mL smooth, highly cohesive, viscous hyaluronic acid filler and its role in facial rejuvenation therapy. *Dermatologic Surgery*, **36** (**3**), 1893–1894.

12 Narins, R.S., Brandt, F., Leyden, J. *et al.* (2003) A randomized, double blind, multicenter comparison of the efficacy and tolerability of Restylane versus Zyplast for the correction of nasolabial folds. *Dermatologic Surgery*, **29**, 588–595.

13 Friedman, P.M., Mafong, E.A., Kauver, A.N. & Geronemus, R.G. (2002) Safety data of injectable nonanimal stabilized hyaluronic acid gel for soft tissue augmentation. *Dermatologic Surgery*, **28**, 491–494.

14 Lowe, N.J., Maxwell, A., Lowe, P. *et al.* (2001) Hyaluronic acid fillers: adverse reactions and skin testing. *Journal of the American Academy of Dermatology*, **45**, 930–933.

15 Hirsh, R. & Stier, M. (2008) Complications of soft tissue augmentation. *Journal of Drugs in Dermatology*, **7** (**9**), 841–845.

16 Brody, H.J. (2005) The use of hyaluronidase in the treatment of granulomatous hyaluronic acid reactions or unwanted hyaluronic acid misplacement. *Dermatologic Surgery*, **31**, 893–897.

17 Jones, D. (2011) Volumizing the face with soft tissue fillers. *Clinics in Plastic Surgery*, **38** (**3**), 379–390.

18 Flaharty, P. (2004) Radiance. *Facial Plastic Surgery*, **20**, 165–169.

19 Carruthers, A. & Carruthers, J. (2008) Evaluation of injectable calcium hydroxylapatite for the treatment of facial lipoatrophy associated with human immunodeficiency virus. *Dermatologic Surgery*, **34**, 1486–1499.

20 Silvers, S.L., Eviatar, J.A., Eschavez, M.I. *et al.* (2006) Prospective, open-label 18-month trial of calcium hydroxylapatite (Radiesse) for facial soft tissue augmentation in patients with human immunodeficiency virus-associated lipoatrophy: one-year durability. *Plastic and Reconstructive Surgery*, **118**, 34S–45S.

21 Day, J.N., Raabe, A., Shiner, A.M. *et al.* (2002) Intradermal polylactic acid (NewFill) for treatment of severe HIV-associated facial lipoatrophy. *HIV Medicine*, **3**, 162.

22 Kates, L.C. & Fitzgerald, R. (2008) Poly-L-lactic acid injection for HIV-associated facial lipoatrophy: treatment principles, case studies, and literature review. *Aesthetic Surgery Journal*, **28** (**4**), 397–403.

23 Fitzgerald, R. & Vleggaar, D. (2011) Facial volume restoration of the aging face with poly-L-lactic acid. *Dermatologic Therapy*, **24** (**1**), 2–27.

24 CL, P. & Jones, D.H. (2006) Liquid injectable silicone for soft tissue augmentation. *Dermatologic Therapy*, **19** (**3**), 159–168.

25 Ellis, L.Z., Cohen, J.L. & High, W. (2012) Granulomatous reaction to silicone injection. *The Journal of Clinical and Aesthetic Dermatology*, **5** (**7**), 44–47.

26 Duffy, D.M. (2002) The silicone conundrum: a battle of anecdotes. *Dermatologic Surgery*, **28**, 590–594.

27 Cohen, S.R. & Holmes, R.E. (2004) Artecoll: a long-lasting injectable wrinkle filler material: report of a controlled, randomized, multicenter clinical trial of 251 subjects. *Plastic and Reconstructive Surgery*, **114**, 964–976.

28 Cohen, S.R., Berner, C.F., Busso, M. *et al.* (2007) Five-year safety and efficacy of a novel polymethylmethacrylate aesthetic soft tissue filler for the correction of nasolabial folds. *Dermatologic Surgery*, **33**, S222–S230.

Index

Fat removal: Invasive and non-invasive body contouring, First Edition. Edited by Mathew M. Avram.
© 2015 John Wiley & Sons, Ltd. Published 2015 by John Wiley & Sons, Ltd.

Printed and bound by CPI Group (UK) Ltd, Croydon, CR0 4YY

16/04/2025

14658829-0001